Iron
The Most
Toxic Metal

Jym Moon, PhD

Foreword by
E.D. Weinberg, PhD

George Ohsawa Macrobiotic Foundation
Chico, California

Other books from the publisher include: *Acid and Alkaline; Basic Macrobiotic Cooking; Essential Ohsawa; Macrobiotics: An Invitation to Health and Happiness; Philosophy of Oriental Medicine; #7 Diet;* and *Zen Macrobiotics.* Contact the publisher at the address below for a complete list of available titles.

Editing by Kathy Keller
Cover design by Carl Campbell
Text layout and design by Carl Ferré

First Edition	2008
Current Edition, minor edits	2011 Nov 7

ISBN 978-0-918860-63-7

Author's Note

My early training was in Nutritional Biochemistry. I worked for about 10 years in the laboratories of Roger J. Williams, who discovered pantothenic acid and was the first to crystallize folic acid and give it its name. The Clayton Foundation Biochemical Institute where I worked is famous for discovering more B-vitamins and their variants than any other single laboratory.

At the time I left the Clayton Foundation, metal toxicology was assuming greater and greater importance. Historically, the time period from 1950 – 2007 might well be referred to as the *Age of Metal Toxicology.* Mercury poisonings were reported in Minimata Bay, Japan in 1953; during the 1960s in Quebec, Canada, the entire Ojibwe nation fell prey to the lethal effects of organic mercury. At the same time, cadmium poisoning resulting in Itai-Itai (Ouch-Ouch) disease was endemic in certain regions of Japan, and manganese was demonstrated to cause a type of amyotropic lateral sclerosis.

In 1980, I decided to return to an academic environment where I could pursue my interest in metal toxicology, and, in 1989, I received a PhD in Biochemical Toxicology from Simon Fraser University in British Columbia. At that time, I was invited to join the British Columbia Hemochromatosis Research Group, where I learned first hand the dangers of over absorption of iron.

For the last 18 years, I have accumulated much of the vast body of scientific information that indicates iron excess is responsible for more sickness and death in North America than any other single factor, including cigarette smoking.

– Jym Moon, PhD, CNS

Foreword

For more than seventy years, the North American public, as well as obdurate bureaucrats, have been enamored with the Popeye-the-Sailor myth, namely, that ingested iron can somehow overcome fatigue and confer strength. During the same time period, however, numerous scientists and medical practitioners have learned to fear rather than praise iron. It is now overwhelmingly apparent that iron loading is a serious risk factor for scores of diseases—an array of cardiovascular disorders; endocrine problems such as diabetes and impotence; neurological ills such as Alzheimer's and Parkinson's; arthritis and osteoporosis; cancers of lung, colon, liver, and skin; nearly all bacterial and fungal infections; and shortened lifespan.

Unfortunately, clever marketing and bureaucratic intransigence have trumped science. It is extremely difficult, if not impossible, for the consumer to select processed foods that have not been deliberately adulterated with troublesome quantities of iron. Finally, a professionally trained toxicologist, Dr. Jym Moon, has assumed the formidable task of dispelling the iron illusion for the public and for the inflexible bureaucrats. Dr. Moon's narrative style is highly appropriate for the intended readers. The book's arguments are strongly reinforced with numerous references to published works of leaders in the field. Thus, Dr. Moon has been able to exclude the use of dubious anecdotal evidence.

Iron—The Most Toxic Metal is a timely, much needed addition for the working desks of leaders in health policy, wellness, and nutrition. Influential persons in such health advocacy groups as arthritis, cancer, diabetes, heart, and neurodegenerative disorders will want copies. The book also will be valuable for officials at all levels of the USDA, FDA, HHS, CDC, NIH, and related units.

Over the long run, scientists generally are optimistic that their work actually can dispel fallacious illusions. Hopefully, Dr. Moon's book will provide the spark that will catalyze the demolishment of the iron myth.

– E.D. Weinberg, PhD
Indiana University
Bloomington, IN

Contents

Chapter 1

A Failed Experiment

Iron Is an Essential Trace Element, but Not a Safe One

Iron is an essential trace element with many important functions in human physiology. In North America, hundreds of thousands of people, predominantly women during menstruation, suffer from "iron deficiency anemia." Although not usually fatal, iron deficiency anemia is reputed to be one of the leading causes of sickness and debility among North American pre-menopausal women.

Iron was one of the first essential trace metals discovered. It has long been known that iron is a critical element for carrying oxygen in the blood. It is the central metal in the oxygen carrying heme complex. Oxygen attaches to heme iron and is transported in this form to various body tissues where it is released to support oxidative metabolism. For this reason, a lack of heme iron results in depressed tissue oxygenation, causing the condition of "iron deficiency anemia."

Because iron deficiency anemia is so common in the target population (menstruating women), public health officials have promoted the addition of iron to many of the most commonly consumed foods, i.e., nutrition supplements, flour, breads, pastas, and breakfast cereals. Despite this practice, iron deficiency anemia remains prevalent in the people who are supposed to be helped by the fortification programs.

In addition to its important function in carrying oxygen, iron is a critical element in numerous enzymes, where it promotes normal metabolism. Iron is also important in the iron-sulfur clusters that facilitate transport of electrons in mitochondria. However, iron deficiency is not known to affect levels of iron-sulfur clusters or enzymes, unless the deficiency is very severe.

Although essential to life, iron is a very toxic metal. Most people are familiar with the highly publicized toxic metals such as lead, mercury, cadmium, manganese, aluminum, and arsenic. However few people know that iron is responsible for a great deal more sickness and death than all of these other toxic metals combined! We have been mesmerized into thinking that iron is somehow different from other metals, simply because it is essential.

Human Iron Balance

The Recommended Dietary Allowance (RDA) for iron for women from 19 years to 50 years is 18 mg/day; for pregnant women it is 27 mg/day, and during lactation, 10 mg/day. The RDA for all other adults is 8 mg/day. The Tolerable Upper Intake Level (UL) for dietary iron is 45 mg/day.

According to the Food and Nutrition Board, one half of ingested iron comes from fortified foods, although this may be an underestimate. Some cereals contain 24 mg iron per 1-cup serving. Most all grain products have varying amounts of iron added—this means virtually all flour, all pastas, all bread, all cereals. Iron supplements commonly sold over the counter contain from 15 mg to around 60 mg iron according to the label-recommended daily intake. It is easy to see how perhaps millions of people in North America are daily consuming more than the UL for iron.

Why are companies allowed to fortify foods with more than the Dietary Reference Intakes (DRIs) in a single serving? What controls are in effect to regulate the amount of iron delivered in food or supplements? Do companies that fortify foods also analyze the food after fortification to determine if the proper amount of iron has been added?

Studies of iron balance in humans have demonstrated that we ordinarily absorb around 15% of the iron that we consume. A person consuming a daily diet containing approximately 15 mg of iron will absorb 1-2 mg. Similarly, approximately 1-2 mg of iron are excreted each day. Children are reported to absorb less iron than adults—around 10%. Pregnant women absorb more—around 17%.

Although only a small percentage of the iron that we consume is absorbed, many factors affect iron absorption. For instance, heme iron is very efficiently absorbed. High heme iron consumption has been correlated with the development of breast cancer. Also, iron absorption can be increased considerably when it is held in the iron 2+ form as it is in the supplements that have combined iron with vitamin C. Iron/vitamin C supplements containing far more than the daily UL for iron are freely sold in spite of their clear danger to human health. Vitron-C®, for instance, contains around 60 mg iron in a single pill as the recommended daily intake. These supplements are very likely the most dangerous "nutritional" supplements ever conceived. Beware!

Iron is a Cumulative Toxin

The inability to excrete iron is the primary problem—we can excrete only around 1.2 mg per day no matter how much we absorb. Once iron has been absorbed in excess of the body's need, it is very difficult to remove it. Much of the excess will be stored in the liver in ferritin. When ferritin is saturated, hemosiderin is released into the liver and can lead to all of the damaging effects of iron to liver cells.

The iron that we consume that is in excess of the amount we absorb is carried through the intestines and excreted in the feces. This iron can be very dangerous because it can exist in free form and generate oxygen radicals resulting in intestinal damage and colon cancer. Colon cancer has been induced in laboratory animals given large excesses of iron. Certain food factors can prevent this kind of damage—in particular phytates that are abundant in plant food.

Iron Fortification of Food

Iron is currently added to most all grain products, including many found in Natural Food stores. In the 1990s, the U.S. Food and Nutrition Board, Institute of Medicine, considered the controversy over iron fortification of food. A number of nutritionists desired to increase the amount of iron added to grain products because "iron-deficiency anemia" was still prevalent in spite of the iron fortification program that had been initiated in the early 1940s.

It was clear even then that the iron-fortification program had failed. The purpose of iron fortification was to eliminate or at least control "iron deficiency anemia" which was prevalent among pre-menopausal women. Unfortunately, the addition of iron to food was unsuccessful. "Iron deficiency anemia," was still endemic among pre-menopausal women in 1990. Instead of acknowledging that the food iron-fortification program had failed, some members of the Food and Nutrition Board desired to increase the amount of iron added to food.

The simple fact is that "iron deficiency anemia" is not a nutritional deficiency disease. There are dozens of very diverse factors that can cause the conditions generally referred to as "iron deficiency anemia." Chronic "iron deficiency anemia," no matter what its origin may be, is a medical problem, not a nutritional problem.

Several iron toxicologists expressed their opinions to the Food and Nutrition Board that iron should be treated like all other metals that accumulate with age in the human body. These specialists suggested that we should minimize iron intake, except under conditions that require additional iron. Otherwise, iron can do serious damage to any and every tissue of the human body. The comments of several of these experts are given here:

1. Randall B. Lauffer, PhD, Harvard Medical School warned the Food and Nutrition Board that his investigations indicated that iron excess may be a primary cause of coronary artery disease. Dr. Lauffer is editor of the first book on iron toxicology, *Iron and Human Disease* (CRC Press, 1992).

2. Dr. J.L. Sullivan, MD, Department of Pathology, University of Florida College of Medicine, provided direct evidence of iron deposits in heart tissue, and showed that stored iron levels are a better predictor of heart disease than is blood cholesterol.

3. E.D. Weinberg, PhD, Indiana University warned that there is an association between iron and hepatocellular carcinoma. He pointed out that iron has been demonstrated to be carcinogenic in laboratory animals, and is known to cause hepatocellular carcinoma in humans.

4. Dr. William Crosby, Director of Hematology at the Chapman Cancer Center in Joplin, Missouri, argued that the Delaney Amendment of 1958 specifically forbids the addition of any substance to food that induces cancer in animals. He suggested that food fortification with iron should be terminated because iron has been shown to cause cancer in both laboratory animals and humans.

5. Baruch S. Blumberg, MD, PhD, Nobel Laureate in Medicine, has spent many years studying the relationship between the hepatitis B virus and liver iron. He warned that high liver iron stores feed the hepatitis B virus, and that this may explain the high incidence of liver cancer found among people infected with the hepatitis B virus.

The Food and Nutrition Board

Since "iron-deficiency anemia" among pre-menopausal women has not been controlled by the food fortification program, and since fatal illnesses due to iron overload are well documented, it seems unreasonable to continue the iron fortification of food. However, the Food and Nutrition Board basically ignored information regarding iron's toxicity, and all grains marketed in North America continue to be "fortified" with iron.

The Food and Nutrition Board, Institute of Medicine, is directly responsible for the food fortification program, and has issued two major statements regarding iron fortification of food.

1. *Iron Deficiency Anemia: Recommended Guidelines for the Prevention, Detection, and Management Among U.S. Children and Women of Childbearing Age.* Committee on the Prevention, Detection, and Management of Iron Deficiency Anemia Among U.S. Children and Women of Childbearing Age. Robert Earl and Catherine E. Woteki, Editors. National Academy Press, Washington, D.C., 1993.

2. *Dietary Reference Intakes for Vitamin A, Vitamin K, Arsenic, Boron, Chromium, Copper, Iodine, Iron, Manganese, Molybdenum, Nickel, Silicon, Vanadium, and Zinc.* National Academy Press, Washington, D.C., 2001.

The most dangerous feature of iron is that it is attracted to, and deposits in, damaged tissue.

In the *Dietary Reference Intakes* (DRIs 2001), the Food and Nutrition Board acknowledged an increased risk for hepatocellular carcinoma in individuals with hereditary hemochromatosis, and reviewed some of the evidence linking iron excess to coronary artery disease. However, there is no mention of the involvement of iron in neuron degeneration caused by iron deposited in the brain. The information linking iron deposits in the brain to Parkinson's, Alzheimer's, and other neurological diseases is compelling. How could the people responsible for the welfare of our entire population have ignored this information?

The Food and Nutrition Board made the following statement in a "Risk Characterization" paragraph stating that the possible cardiovascular and hepatic hazards make it "prudent to recommend that men and postmenopausal women avoid iron supplements and highly fortified foods." However, there was still no mention of the neurological risks. Also, because most all grains continue to be fortified with varying amounts of iron, the Food and Nutrition Board didn't offer any way for people to avoid these "highly fortified foods," nor has there been any attempt to inform people that they may be harmed by these foods.

The Biochemical Basis of Iron Toxicity

Under healthy circumstances, iron is tightly bound to organic components. This binding is referred to as chelation. Chelation prevents iron from redox cycling. Hemoglobin and myoglobin are the most abundant mammalian hemoprotiens, but there are also cytochromes and enzymes that utilize iron. In addition, iron is present in iron-sulfur clusters that are important in electron transfer reactions.

However, when present in excess, iron poses a threat to cells and tissues. Iron exists as ferrous iron, Fe(II), or ferric iron, Fe(III). Free iron can be oxidized from ferrous iron to ferric iron, and reduced from ferric iron to ferrous iron. This is known as redox cycling. When iron redox cycles, oxygen radicals are generated. The resulting superoxide and hydroxyl radicals damage cell structures.

Iron Excess Worsens Chronic Illness

Iron can accumulate in free form in any body tissue under conditions of iron overload. That is why iron excess causes such a wide variety of illnesses.

The most dangerous feature of iron is that it is attracted to, and deposits in, damaged tissue. Thus, the neurofibrillary tangles of Alzheimer's, the substantia nigra of Parkinson's, the atherosclerotic plaques of coronary artery disease, the inflamed joints of arthritis, the pancreatic islet cells of adult-onset diabetics all display increased levels of free iron. There is no way to tell whether the iron initiates the disease or if the diseased tissue attracts the iron which then exacerbates the condition. But either way, free iron in any body tissue is dangerous.

As stated earlier, nearly every individual in North America displays some manifestation of iron poisoning with advancing age. Here is a brief list—these and other diseases will be discussed at length in the following chapters.

- **Neurological Degeneration: Parkinson's & Alzheimer's**
  o The brain is a major target for excess iron.

- o Accumulation of iron in brain tissue either causes, or contributes to, neurological diseases such as Parkinsonism and Alzheimer's disease.
- **Cancer:** Iron is a powerful carcinogen.
  - o Excess iron is a well-documented cause of hepatocellular carcinoma.
  - o Elevated levels of iron predispose to breast cancer.
  - o Animals fed iron excesses develop colon cancer, believed to be the result of free radical generation by unabsorbed iron.
- **Heart Disease:**
  - o Excess iron accumulates in the heart and arteries.
  - o Free iron as found in heart and arteries may provoke arterial damage.
- **Diabetes:**
  - o In hereditary hemochromatosis, excess iron accumulates in the pancreas where it disrupts insulin secretion and causes adult-onset diabetes.
  - o Iron deposits are found in pancreatic islet cells in people with adult-onset diabetes.
- **Joint Inflammation/Arthritis:** Iron is found in free form in arthritic joints.
- **Osteoporosis:** People with transfusion siderosis develop osteoporosis at a very young age; iron accumulation in bone causes osteopenia and osteoporosis.
- **Pituitary Function:** People with hereditary iron overload may have "hypogonadotrophic hypogonadism"—infertility due to iron accumulation in the pituitary gland.
- **Sperm Damage:** Iron overload diseases are uniformly associated with sperm damage.
- **Sexual dysfunction:**
  - o Hypogonadotrophic hypogonadism & infertility.
  - o Sperm and egg DNA damage.
- **Eye diseases:** age related macular degeneration (AMD).
- **Kidney damage:** hypertension.

- **Hearing Loss.**
- **Cerebrovascular accidents:** stroke.

Chapter 2

A Brief History

Introduction

The current climate of opinion in North America places iron on a pedestal. Contemporary thinking of people in general can be summarized: "Iron is essential and will restore health and vitality and overcome that 'run down' feeling." Nutritionists contribute to this misconception by insisting that "iron-deficiency anemia" is the number one nutritional deficiency disease in North America, in spite of the fact that there is a great deal of conflicting information. This misconception is based on nutritional surveys that do not evaluate the health status of individuals with lowered hemoglobin count or low transferrin loading. We will discuss this later.

It is easy to understand how such a misunderstanding has developed. From earliest times, it has been recognized that women who lose blood during menstruation may develop pale skin and weakness. Iron deficiency anemia may result as a natural consequence of blood loss during menstruation. Various iron-rich foods have been recommended at different periods throughout history.

In actual fact, "iron-deficiency anemia" is not that common. Menstruation does not cause iron deficiency anemia in the vast majority of women. Even though hemoglobin levels and transferrin loading may be temporarily lowered, women who menstruate simply absorb more iron from their food. Thus, if "iron deficiency anemia" does temporarily manifest, it is rapidly counteracted by greater iron absorption.

One feature of anemia is the development of paleness of the skin, with a slight bluish-green tint. The condition is referred to as *chlorosis* (from the Greek word for green). In 1893, Ralph Stockman, a lecturer at the School of Medicine in Edinburgh, Scotland, showed that the hemoglobin levels in chlorotic women were low, and could be raised by iron supplementation, causing the skin to return to its normal slightly pink color.

1929: From Popeye to Geritol®

Popeye entered the scene in 1929 and soon became a true American hero. By consuming a can of spinach, Popeye developed super strength and rescued his beloved Olive Oyl from his archenemy, Bluto. As advertising and public mentality would have it, the iron in spinach invigorated Popeye, and he could do virtually anything. In actual fact, spinach is not a good source of iron because the iron in spinach is not readily available for absorption.

With Popeye, the notion developed that iron could somehow overcome fatigue and confer strength on anyone who took it. This idea was well ingrained in the North American population by the 1950s when the J.B. Williams Company devised a marketing scheme to sell their iron supplement known as Geritol®. Geritol® was extensively promoted with the claim that taking it would give a person great strength. Soon the name Geritol®, like Popeye, became a household name and became synonymous with strength, health, and vitality. Iron-fortified foods and iron supplements were well established as an integral part of life for everyone in North America—a true cornerstone for health.

The Federal Trade Commission challenged the promotion of Geritol® as a vitality-conferring supplement and, after more than a decade of court cases, finally forced the makers of Geritol® to cease false advertising. However, because Popeye and Geritol® had become household names, the North American population was indoctrinated to believe that iron supplements can really confer strength and vitality. (Refer to Lauffer 1993, pp 33-42 for a review of the Geritol® scam.)

1941: Iron Adulteration of Food

By the early 1930s, a number of serious illnesses that had plagued humans for centuries had been shown to be vitamin deficiency diseases. Scurvy was due to a deficiency of vitamin C, pellagra to a niacin deficiency, beriberi to a thiamin deficiency, and rickets to a vitamin D deficiency. By the end of the 1930s, these illnesses were virtually eliminated in North America through vitamin usage. There was ample evidence that addition of these vitamins to various foods and supplements would be safe and effective. Thus, it was hoped that addition of iron to dietary staples would similarly eliminate the chlorosis of menstruation.

The first Nationwide Food Consumption Survey was conducted in 1936-1937. Following this survey, President Franklin Roosevelt called for a National Nutrition Conference in 1941. The first RDAs were established, and the FDA set the first standards for enrichment of food. Iron and the B-complex vitamins thiamin, riboflavin, and niacin were added to processed grain products with the claim that the additions were simply restoring levels of these nutrients that had been removed during processing of the grains.

1969: The FDA Increased Iron in Food

The White House Conference on Food, Nutrition, and Health held in 1969 conducted formal hearings on the food fortification program. "Iron deficiency anemia" was touted as the Number One nutritional deficiency disease in North America. The American Bakers Association and the Millers National Federation made a formal proposal to the FDA to quadruple the amount of iron in wheat flour and bakery products. On April 1, 1970 the FDA proposed to triple the quantity of iron added to milled grains. (Did the FDA actually intend to pull an April fool's joke, or is the date simply coincidental?)

To increase the level of iron added to grains would likely be a slow-death warrant to the 1.5 million people in North America with hereditary hemochromatosis, and would have serious consequences for the 37 million North Americans who are heterozygous for the hemochromatosis gene. Why? In order to alleviate chlorosis of menstruation in the 2 or 3 million women who periodically develop "iron-deficiency anemia?" What kind of reasoning is that? Why not provide iron-fortified foods as a special food for women of childbearing age? Universal iron fortification of milled grain products forces everyone who wants to eat bread, cereals, crackers, and pastas to consume the added iron whether they need it or not, and even if it kills them!

Dr. Margaret Ann Krikker and Dr. William Crosby led the group of 174 physicians who opposed the proposal to increase iron fortification, and recommended that iron fortification be terminated. By comparison, 16 physicians—along with the American Bakers Association and the Millers National Federation—endorsed the proposal.

Lauffer (1993, pp 62-63) summarized the situation:

> Those physicians opposed to fortification thought they were victorious in 1977-1978 when FDA commissioner, Donald Kennedy, who clearly saw the problems, struck down the proposal. In the *Federal Register* of August 29, 1978, Commissioner Kennedy wrote: "There is insufficient evidence that the augmentation in iron-fortified bread would ameliorate the condition of those who need iron…There are no adequate studies showing the safety of the increased levels of iron in bread…Because of the findings and conclusions above, the augmentation of iron-fortification of bread…should not be approved."

Although the attempts to increase the amount of iron added to foods by 3-fold failed, the FDA went ahead and mandated a 50 percent increase in the iron content of flour, contrary to Commissioner Kennedy's recommendations. Millers and bakers held onto their precious position of providing vigor and vitality for all. (Refer to Lauffer 1993, pp 61-73 for a more complete discussion, and references to Federal Register documentation of the FDA actions.)

1970 – 2007: Beyond Geritol®

When it was discovered that vitamin C can enhance absorption of iron, manufacturers of nutrition supplements took the next logical step, combining iron with vitamin C. This gave rise to supplements such as Vitron-C®, which contains around 60 mg iron combined with 200 mg vitamin C. The name suggests that Vitron-C® gives vitality to those who consume it. The label on Vitron-C® states that it contains 365% of the Daily Value, which is more than 800% of the RDA for men and postmenopausal women. It even exceeds the Tolerable Upper Intake Level (UL) of 45 mg/day.

In compliance with an FDA ruling of January 15, 1997 (62 FR 2218), the label on Vitron-C® warns that children should not have access: "Accidental overdose of iron-containing products is the leading cause of fatal poisoning in children under 6. Keep this product out of the reach of children. In case of accidental overdose, call a doctor or poison control center immediately." The FDA ruling covers all supplements with 30 mg or more iron per dosage unit with the exception of supplements containing the elemental form of iron (iron carbonyl), which the FDA considered to be less toxic than iron salts.

Even though it was well-known in 1997, when the FDA was formulating warning labels for iron supplements, that people with hereditary hemochromatosis are endangered by iron-containing supplements, there is no warning that anyone other than young children might be harmed by taking the supplements.

Hereditary Iron Overload

Hemochromatosis is one of the first iron storage diseases recognized. Although described in 1865 (Trousseau 1865), it was not until 1935 when Sheldon published the first monograph on the condition that hemochromatosis began to emerge as a coherent hereditary clinical entity. Sheldon's monograph was based on his analysis of 311 cases that had been recorded at that time. In 1955, Finch and Finch added 80 of their own patients and reviewed another 707 histologically proven cases that had been reported since the publication of Sheldon's monograph. Hemochromatosis was defined as a general increase in body iron stores with associated tissue damage.

The organs most frequently damaged by iron overload are the heart, liver, pancreas, brain, and pituitary gland. Soon it was recognized that this condition is inherited (as first suggested by Sheldon), and it became known as hereditary hemochromatosis.

Hereditary hemochromatosis is an inherited condition in which too much iron is absorbed. Because there is no physiologic mechanism for excreting iron, the excess accumulates in various tissues in ferritin—a tube-like protein structure that encases the iron—thereby preventing redox cycling. However, once the ability to store iron is exceeded, hemosiderin is released with consequent iron redox cycling and tissue damage. Hereditary hemochromatosis is the most common genetically transferred disease among people of northern European descent. Approximately 0.5% of North Americans are homozygous for the hemochromatosis gene, and approximately 10% are carriers.

Transfusion Siderosis

Blood transfusions are occasionally needed to control other hematological disorders. Among these conditions, the thalassemias are best known. Thalassemias are inherited disorders in which the body lacks the ability to synthesize normal heme. Some populations—in particular people living around the Mediterranean Sea (people of Greek and Italian descent)—ß-thalassemia is not uncommon, affecting as many as 1 in 400 people. The disease also is quite prevalent in the Near East, the Middle East, India, Southeast Asia, and South China (Weinberg 2004, p 13). Because each unit of blood contains approximately 0.2 g of iron, these patients soon become overloaded with iron. Unlike the circumstance in hemochromatosis, phlebotomy is not an option for iron removal. Iron chelators such as deferrioxamine have been used intravenously. On November 9, 2005, the FDA approved the first oral drug for chronic iron overload. The drug is known as Exjade® (deferasirox), manufactured by Novartis Pharmaceutical Corporation, Stein, Switzerland.

Hemosiderosis Among the Bantus

In 1953 Walker and Arvidsson reported a condition of iron overload among South African Bantus that was caused by excessive iron ingestion. The condition had been previously reported in 1928 (Strachan 1929), but the cause of the illness wasn't investigated in detail until the report of Walker and Arvidsson (1953). The Bantus were brewing their alcoholic beverage in iron pots, and were getting from 50 to 100 mg iron per day from this source. The condition was later described as hemosiderosis to distinguish it from the hereditary condition of hemochromatosis where excess iron is absorbed even from relatively low iron ingestion. The condition has now been observed in nearly all sub-Saharan African countries and may affect up to 10% of the population (Bothwell et al. 1979).

The discoveries of these iron overload diseases (hereditary hemochromatosis, hemosiderosis, and ß-thalassemia) demonstrated that iron overload can arise as a result of several circumstances: from hereditary overabsorption of iron; from too much iron in the diet; or from multiple blood transfusions. However, the explanation for the vast array of illnesses that can result from iron overload remained a mystery until Halliwell and Gutteridge (1984) demonstrated generation of oxygen radicals by iron in biological systems.

1981: Iron Misregulation and Ischemic Heart Disease

Hemochromatosis was first described in 1865, and hemosiderosis was observed among South African Bantus in 1928. However, prior to the 1980s, it was generally believed that iron was not very toxic. Hemochromatosis was thought to be a rare condition, and the circumstance among the Bantus was simply a condition of consuming exceptionally large amounts of iron contained in an alcoholic beverage. Iron absorption and toxicity is enhanced by alcohol. We will discuss the important relationship between alcoholic cirrhosis and iron in more detail later.

The potential for iron to be toxic to large numbers of people was first suggested by Jerome Sullivan (1981) in his now classic article, "Iron and the sex difference in heart disease risk." Sullivan hypothesized that the menstrual loss of iron is the primary factor protecting premenopausal women from ischemic heart disease. This marks a very important turning point in the developing science of iron toxicology.

1982: Formation of The Hemochromatosis Research Foundation

By 1982, it became evident that hemochromatosis is more than a medical curiosity. In fact, the hereditary form of hemochromatosis was demonstrated to affect millions of people worldwide, and is the most common inherited condition that disposes to illness. In 1982, The Hemochromatosis Research Foundation was established under the leadership of Dr. Margaret Krikker. The Hemochromatosis Research Foundation has been absorbed by the Iron Disorders Institute and is directed by Cheryl Garrison.

1984: Iron Can Redox Cycle in Biological Systems

It wasn't until 1984 when Halliwell and Gutteridge demonstrated oxygen radical generation by iron in biological systems that iron's potential for toxicity began to be appreciated. This discovery provided a mechanism that could explain why iron can be damaging to so many organs, and is an unusually important milestone in iron toxicology. We will discuss the role of iron in generating oxygen radicals in a later chapter. By now, the literature dealing with iron toxicology is vast, but public education is lacking primarily due to the very vocal nutritionists who wish to foist iron-adulterated foods on developing countries.

1988: The First International Conference on Hemochromatosis

The First International Conference on Hemochromatosis was held by the New York Academy of Sciences on April 27-29, 1987 in New York, New York. The conference proceedings were published in Volume 526, Annals of the New York Academy of Sciences (Weintraub et al. 1988).

1992: Iron Toxicology Became Firmly Established

Finally, in 1992 with the publication of *Iron and Human Disease* (Lauffer, ed 1992), iron joined ranks with the other toxic metals that bioaccumulate with age: lead, mercury, cadmium, manganese, thallium, silver, platinum, aluminum, and arsenic. By now, iron toxicology has outdone all of the other toxic metals and is the most extensive branch of metal toxicology.

1992 – 2007: Continuing Contributions to Iron Toxicology

The information gathered in the years since iron toxicology became established as the most extensive branch of metal toxicology will be discussed later in the chapters dealing with each of these topics.

Table I. Some Important Dates in Iron Toxicology

Year	Event	Reference
1936	Dreyfus reported lung cancer in two siblings who inhaled iron dust while polishing watch screws with iron oxide.	Dreyfus J.
1941	Iron adulteration of milled grains was initiated in North America to ensure that everyone receive enough iron.	Refer to Lauffer RB. (1993), pp 60-63.
1946	Discovery of transferrin.	Schade A, Caroline L.

1952	The first siderophore, ferrichrome, was crystallized from a rust fungus, Ustilago sphaerogena.	Neilands JB.
1953	Hemosiderosis in South African Bantus brewing alcoholic beverage in iron pots. From 50-100 mg iron caused hemosiderosis/liver cancer.	Walker ARP, Arvidsson UB; and Bothwell TH.
1961	The complete structure of ferrichrome, the first siderophore discovered, was announced.	Emery TF, Neilands JB
1966	The first article indicating that iron withholding could defend against infectious diseases.	Weinberg ED.
1969	The FDA proposed to triple the amount of iron added to fortified foods.	Refer to Lauffer RB (1993) pp 60-63.
1981	Jerome Sullivan hypothesized that excess iron is the primary factor responsible for the higher incidence of ischemic heart disease among men as compared to women.	Sullivan JL.
1982	Margaret Krikker announced the formation of the Hemochromatosis Research Foundation.	Krikker MA
1982	The Canadian Hemochromatosis Society, initiated by Marie Warder in 1978, was incorporated in 1982.	Refer to Garrison C, ed. (2001, pp 255-56)
1982	Iron Overload Diseases (IOD) was established by Roberta Crawford.	Refer to Garrison C, ed. (2001, pp 255-56)
1984	Halliwell and Gutteridge demonstrated iron-catalyzed oxygen radical generation in living systems.	Halliwell B, Gutteridge JMC.
1988	The First International Conference on Hemochromatosis.	Weintraub LR, Edwards CQ, Krikker M.
1992	Iron and Human Disease, the first full-length book on iron toxicity, was published. This publication marks the coming of age of Iron Toxicology. Iron joined ranks with other metals that accumulate with age: mercury, lead, cadmium, aluminum, manganese, thallium, silver, platinum, and arsenic.	Lauffer RB, ed.

1996	Discovery of two HFE gene mutations that can result in hereditary hemochromatosis.	Feder JN, et al.
2001	Hepcidin was discovered.	Parks CH, Valore EV, Waring AJ, Ganz T.
2006	Dunaief identified iron accumulation as a probable cause of age-related macular degeneration.	Dunaief JL.
2007	Tappel hypothesized that epidemiological evidence linking red meat consumption to numerous human illnesses may be due to the presence of heme iron in red meat.	Tappel A.

Table 2. Some Books on Iron Toxicology

Date	Title/Publisher	Author(s)
1935	*Haemochromatosis*. London: Oxford Univ. Press	Sheldon JH.
1964	*Hemochromatosis and Hemosiderosis*. Springfield, IL: Charles C. Thomas	MacDonald RA.
1984	*The Bronze Killer*. Delta, B.C. Canada: Imperani Publishers	Warder M
1987	*Iron and Infection*. Chichester, New York, Brisbane, Toronto, Singapore: John Wiley & Sons	Bullen JJ, Griffiths E.
1991	*Iron and Your Health: Facts and Fallacies*. Boca Raton, Boston, Ann Arbor: CRC Press	Emery TF.
1992	*Iron and Human Disease*. Boca Raton, Ann Arbor, London, Tokyo: CRC Press	Lauffer RB, ed.
1993	*Iron and Your Heart*. New York: St. Martin's Press: New York	Lauffer RB.
1994	*Secondary Iron Overload*. London: W.B. Saunders Company Ltd.	Pippard MJ.
1999	*The Iron Time Bomb*. San Dimas, CA: Bill Sardi	Sardi, B.
2001	*Guide to Hemochromatosis*. Nashville: Cumberland House	The Iron Disorders Institute. Garrison C, ed.

2000	*The Iron Elephant, 2nd edition.* Glyndon, MD: Vida Publishing, Inc.	Crawford R.
2002	*The Iron Factor of Aging.* Tucson: Fenestra Books	Facchini FS.
2003	*The Iron Disorders Institute Guide to Anemia.* Nashville: Cumberland House	The Iron Disorders Institute. Garrison C, ed.
2004	*Exposing the Hidden Dangers of Iron.* Nashville: Cumberland House	Weinberg ED.

REFERENCES

Bothwell TH, Charlton AW, Cook JD, Finch CA. 1979. *Iron Metabolism in Man.* Oxford: Blackwell Scientific Publications.

Crawford R. 2000. *The Iron Elephant.* Glyndon, MD: Vida Publishing, Inc.

Dreyfus J. 1936. Lung carcinoma among siblings who have inhaled dust containing iron oxides during their youth. Clin Med. 30:256-60.

Dunaief JL. 2006. Iron induced oxidative damage as a potential factor in age-related macular degeneration: the Cogan Lecture. Invest Ophthalmol Vis Sci. 47:4660-664.

Emery T, Neilands JB. 1961. Structure of the ferrichrome compounds. J Am Chem Soc. 83:1626.

Emery TF. 1991. *Iron and Your Health: Facts and Fallacies.* Boca Raton, Boston, Ann Arbor: CRC Press.

Facchini FS. 2002. *The Iron Factor of Aging.* Tucson, AZ: Fenestra Books.

Feder JN, Gnirke A, Thomas Z, Tsuchihashi Z, Ruddy DA, Basava A, Dormishian G, Domingo R Jr, Ellis MC, Fullan A, Hinton LM, Jones NL, Kimmel BE, Kronmal GS, Lauer P, Lee VK, Loeb DB, Mapa FA, McClelland E, Meyer NC, Mintier GA, Moeller N, Moore T, Morikang EB, Prass CE, Quintana L, Stames SM, Schatzman RC, Brunke KJ, Drayana DT, Risch NJ, Bacon BR, Wolff RK. 1996. A novel MHC class 1-like gene is mutated in patients with hereditary haemochromatosis. Nat Genet. 13(4):399-408.

Finch SC, Finch CA. 1955. Medicine (Baltimore). 34:384-430.

Garrison C, ed. 2001. *Guide to Hemochromatosis.* Nashville: Cumberland House.

——— 2003. *The Iron Disorders Institute Guide to Anemia.* Nashville: Cumberland House.

Halliwell B, Gutteridge JMC. 1984. Oxygen toxicity, oxygen radicals, transition metals and disease. Biochem J. 219:1.

Krikker MA. 1982. A foundation for hemochromatosis (letter). Ann Intern Med. 97:782-83.

Lauffer RB, ed. 1992. *Iron and Human Disease.* Boca Raton, Ann Arbor, London, Tokyo: CRC Press.

Lauffer RB. 1993. *Iron and Your Heart.* New York: St Martin's Press.

MacDonald RA. 1964. *Hemochromatosis and Hemosiderosis.* Springfield, IL: Charles C Thomas Press.

Neilands JB. 1952. A crystalline organo-iron pigment from a rust fungus, *Ustilago sphaerogena.* 74:4846.

Parks CH, Valore EV, Waring AJ, Ganz T. 2001. Hepcidin, a urinary antimicrobial peptide synthesized in the liver. 278(11):7806-816.

Pippard MJ. 1994. *Secondary Iron Overload.* London: WB Saunders Company Ltd.

Sardi B. 1999. *The Iron Time Bomb.* San Dimas, CA: Bill Sardi.

Shade AL, Caroline L. 1946. An iron binding component in human blood plasma. Science. 104:340-41.

Sheldon JH. 1935. *Haemochromatosis.* London: Oxford Univ Press.

Strachan AS. 1929. MD Thesis. University of Glasgow.

Sullivan JL. 1981. Iron and the sex difference in heart disease risk. The Lancet. pp 1293-94.

Tappel A. 2007. Heme of consumed red meat can act as a catalyst of oxidative damage and could initiate colon, breast and prostate cancers, heart disease and other diseases. Med Hypothesis. 68(3):562-4.

Trousseau A. 1865. Clinique Méd de l'Hôtel de Paris (2d edit). 2:663-98.

Walker ARP, Arvidsson UB. 1953. Iron 'overload' in South African Bantu. J R Soc Trop Med Hyg. 47:536-48.

Weinberg ED. 1966 Roles of metallic ions in host-parasite interactions. Bacteriological Reviews. 30:1336-51.

——— 2004. *Exposing the Hidden Dangers of Iron.* Nashville: Cumberland House.

Weintraub LR, Edwards CQ, Krikker M. 1988. Hemochromatosis. Proceedings of the First International Conference. Ann NY Acad Sci. Volume 256.

Chapter 3

How Much Iron?

Level of Fortification

In the 2001 issue of *Dietary Reference Intakes* (DRIs) for Iron, the Panel on Micronutrients of the Food and Nutrition Board writes, "The median dietary intake of iron is approximately 16 to 18 mg per day for men and 12 mg/day for women." Let us take a look at these estimates.

Apparently, there is a great deal of freedom as to the amount of iron that can be added to food. The 2001 DRIs states, "Some fortified cereals contain as much as 24 mg of iron per 1-cup serving." (Food and Nutrition Board 2001, p 356). We will use this value to make an estimate as to how much iron some people are actually consuming.

The estimated intakes of iron used by the Panel on Micronutrients were based on the assumption that iron-supplemented food contains the actual amount stated on the label. P. Whittaker and colleagues (2002) from the FDA analyzed twenty-nine cereals for iron content.

"When the labeled value was compared to the assayed value for iron content, 21 of the 29 cereals were 120% or more of the label value and 8 were 150% or more of the label value. This gives us an approximate estimate that fortified cereals contain around 1.3 times as much iron as the label states."

Now let us make an estimate as to how much iron a person might consume from iron-fortified cereal. Whittaker and colleagues have already done this for us, so let us accept their findings in order to come up with some estimate of how much iron we really are consuming.

"Serving size quantities were estimated in 72 adults who regularly ate cereal. The median analyzed serving size was 47 g for females, and 61 g for males with a combined median of 56 g as compared to the label value of 30 g. For adults, the amount of cereal actually consumed was approximately 200% of the labeled serving size."

Because the one-cup serving of cereal cited in the DRIs provides, according to the label, 24 mg of iron, and cereal eaters usually eat around two cups, that cereal has provided 48 mg of iron, assuming the label is accurate.

Now, let us consider that the cereal may actually contain 130% of the label-stated amount, as found by Whittaker. A person eating a couple of cups of cereal could be ingesting as much as 62 mg iron! This is well above the Tolerable Upper Intake Level (UL) of 45 mg/day. Let us hope that cereal eaters do not also take an iron containing supplement!

Labels are Misleading

Labels on iron supplements are, according to guidelines established by the FDA, expressed as percent Daily Value (%DV).

Unfortunately, labeling as %DV is very misleading in the case of iron. The "Daily Value" for labeling for iron is 18 mg iron, and has nothing to do with the human need for iron. The Recommended Dietary Allowance (RDA) for adult males and post-menopausal

	EAR	RDA	DV
Men (19 years and older)	6 mg/day	8 mg/day	18 mg/day
Women (51 years and older)	5 mg/day	8 mg/day	18 mg/day
Women (19 to 50 years)	8.1 mg/day	18 mg/day	18 mg/day
• **EAR** = Estimated Average Requirement • **RDA** = Recommended Dietary Allowance • **DV** = Daily Value used for labeling purposes			

women is 8 mg iron. Therefore, a supplement that provides 18 mg iron supplies 225% of the RDA for these people. However, the label states that it is only 100% of the DV. Because the amount of iron a person needs does not depend on the caloric intake, labels on iron-containing supplements should state the percent of the RDA or Estimated Average Requirement (EAR), *not* the %DV.

To confuse things even more, some supplements do not express the iron content, but express, for instance, the iron fumarate content. The labeling on Vitron-C® illustrates this. The label lists the amount of ferrous fumarate (not the amount of iron). According to the label, 200 mg ferrous fumarate provides 325% of the DV for iron. It contains 712% of the RDA for adults other than premenopausal women.

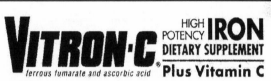

VITRON·C
ferrous fumarate and ascorbic acid®

HIGH POTENCY **IRON**
DIETARY SUPPLEMENT
Plus Vitamin C

DIRECTIONS: Adults – one or two tablets daily or as directed by a physician. Tablets should be swallowed whole. Do not exceed recommended dosage.

WARNING: Accidental overdose of iron-containing products is a leading cause of fatal poisoning in children under 6. Keep this product out of reach of children. In case of accidental overdose, call a doctor or poison control center immediately.

Supplement Facts

Serving Size 1 Tablet

Amount Per Tablet	% Daily Value
Vitamin C (ascorbic acid) 125mg	200%
Iron (ferrous fumarate) 200mg	365%

OTHER INGREDIENTS: cellulose, croscarmellose sodium, iron oxide, magnesium stearate, microcrystalline cellulose, mono and di-glycerides, polyethylene glycol, polyvinyl alcohol, sodium ascorbate, talc, titanium dioxide,

WARNING: The treatment of any anemic condition should be under the advice and supervision of a physician. As oral iron products interfere with absorption of oral tetracycline antibiotics, these products should not be taken within two hours of each other. As with any dietary supplement, if you are pregnant or nursing a baby, seek the advice of a health professional before using this product.

Store at room temperature, 15°-30°C (59°-86°F).

)UESTI ONS? Call 1-800-344-7239 or write to Consumer Affairs at the address below.

Distributed by:
INSIGHT Pharmaceuticals Corp.
Blue Bell, PA 19422-2726

Visit us at our website
www.insightpharma.com

By comparison, the label on Ferro-Sequels® states that the product contains 50 mg of iron (derived from ferrous fumarate). The 50 mg of iron in Ferro-Sequels® is 625% the RDA, and even exceeds the UL (Tolerable Upper Intake Level), but the label indicates that it contains 277% of the Daily Value.

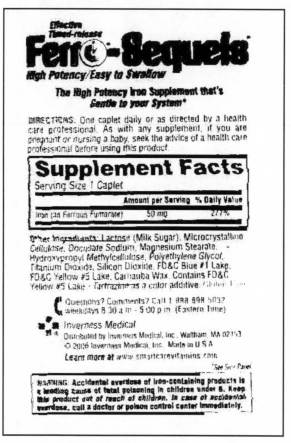

Conclusion: It is not possible to determine from the label what percentage of the RDA is actually contained in any particular iron supplement. A similar circumstance is found for iron-fortified cereals. Determining the amount of iron in cereals is even more difficult, because the actual weight of iron is not given on the label—only the %DV is given. Labels for iron should contain both the actual amount of iron per serving, and the %RDA, or %EAR.

Choose Your Poison

The chemical nature of the iron is important. Iron must be in the divalent form (Fe^{2+}) for efficient absorption, so most of the iron that is used in fortification is Fe^{2+}. However, very fine iron powder, where iron is in the neutral state (Fe^0), is apparently also permitted and used. Some of the other forms of iron used for supplementation include iron(II) oxide, iron(II) fumarate, iron(II) sulfate, and carbonyl iron (Fe^0). The 1993 report on Iron Deficiency Anemia of the Food and Nutrition Board lists 7 different kinds of iron(III) and 7 different kinds of iron(II) compounds that are approved. (Refer to Table 5, page 84 for a list of 20 iron compounds currently approved by the FDA.)

An FDA-approved red food coloring is apparently a mixture of iron(II) and iron(III) oxides. The FDA has also approved two iron "flavor enhancers"—iron chloride and iron sulfate. It is certain that no one knows how much of these "flavor enhancers" is being used, nor what foods they are used in.

Some of the newer additions to the list of iron additives are iron(II) EDTA, iron-choline citrate complex, and iron(II) ascorbate.

Whittaker and colleagues (2001) from the FDA reported on the genotoxicity of various forms of iron. "We found that elemental and salt forms of Fe, including compounds used in dietary supplements and for food fortification, induced mutagenic responses in L5178Y mouse lymphoma cells.... Exposure of mouse lymphoma cells to Fe^0, Fe^{2+}, and Fe^{3+} resulted in the induction of mutagenic responses with likely different mechanisms of iron metabolism."

Heme Iron and Human Disease

Heme iron refers to the iron that is found in red meat. Heme iron is much more efficiently absorbed than most other forms of iron. A recent article by A. Tappel (2007) from the University of California, Davis, presents a summary of the role of heme iron in a variety of diseases.

"Dietary epidemiological studies indicate correlations between the consumption of red meat and/or processed meat and cancer of the colon, rectum, stomach, pancreas, bladder, endometrium, ovaries, prostate, breast, and lung; heart disease; rheumatoid arthritis; type 2 diabetes; and Alzheimer's disease. The correlation of all these major diseases with dietary red meat indicates the presence of factors in red meat that damage biological components. This hypothesis will focus on the biochemistry of heme compounds and their oxidative processes" (Tappel 2007).

Iron, Lung Cancer, and Vitamin C

When iron(II) is combined with vitamin C, the iron is very efficiently absorbed—perhaps as efficiently as is heme iron. This is the basis for the more recently formulated iron supplements that are currently being sold in North America. As iron(II)-vitamin C, 40 or 50% of the ingested iron may be absorbed, compared to the ordinary 15% or less.

The Iowa Women's Health Study (Lee and Jacobs 2005) addressed the question of "Interaction among heme iron, zinc, and supplemental vitamin C intake on the risk of lung cancer." Increased heme iron intake was associated with increased lung cancer. The higher the vitamin C intake, the greater the association between heme iron and lung cancer. A note of caution to smokers who think vitamin C will act as an antioxidant and protect them. The antioxidant properties of vitamin C are compromised, and it carries a powerful pro-oxidant into the body!

Genetically Modified Iron-Accumulating Grains

In recent years, genetically-modified iron-accumulating strains of rice, wheat, and corn have been developed (Gura 1999), and are probably being used. Their intended use is in developing countries where iron deficiency is believed to be common. Whenever these "naturally iron-enriched" grains are used, they should be clearly marked. Unfortunately, there are currently no labeling regulations for them.

Intervention by genetically-modified iron-rich grains needs to be very carefully evaluated. The Somali nomads are one group that is targeted as needing iron supplementation. They consume a milk-based diet—one that is considered to be severely deficient in iron. The hemoglobin levels of Somali men indicate that—by comparison with medical standards for Caucasian males—the Somalis have "iron-deficiency anemia." However, even with low hemoglobin levels, they are very vigorous people and do not suffer clinical symptoms of anemia.

"Iron-deficiency" is believed to result in reduced resistance to infection. Higher rates of infection among children have been clearly demonstrated in several populations throughout the world. However, this observation may not apply to all populations. In 1978, a group of researchers reported results of a very interesting experiment on the incidence of infection among "iron-deficient" and iron-supplemented Somali men (Murray et al. 1978).

"The incidence of infection was studied in 137 iron-deficient Somali men, 67 of whom were treated with placebo and 71 with iron. Seven episodes of infection occurred in the placebo group and 36 in the group treated with iron; these 36 episodes included activation of pre-existing malaria, brucellosis, and tuberculosis. This difference suggested that host defense against these infections was better during iron deficiency than during iron repletion."

At the end of 30 days, the men who received the iron tablets showed a 50% increase of blood hemoglobin. "Iron-deficiency" in these Somali men protects them from infection. Because infectious diseases are the primary cause of death among the Somali, dietary intervention must be carefully evaluated.

Women of Childbearing Age

Women of childbearing age are not as susceptible to iron toxicity as are men and post-menopausal women. In fact, these women are the target group for iron deficiency. Iron supplementation may be necessary. The reason should be apparent: Monthly loss of blood protects women from iron accumulation, but makes them susceptible to iron deficiency.

However, even menstruating women should be very cautious in using iron-containing supplements. The vast majority of menstruating women do not develop iron deficiency anemia. They may develop transient anemia, but this is quickly reversed because they naturally absorb more iron from the diet. The Food and Nutrition Board (1993) estimated the incidence of "iron deficiency anemia" among women of childbearing age to be 4 to10 percent. Even this estimate may be too high, because it is based on national surveys that do not take into consideration the occurrence of the symptoms of iron deficiency.

It would be wise for any woman who suspects that she is in need of iron to consult a physician before taking any iron supplement. Diagnosis of iron deficiency anemia should be based on several blood measurements including: hematocrit, hemoglobin content, transferrin binding, and serum ferritin.

Acute Iron Poisoning

According to the FDA, accidental iron overdose is the most common cause of poisoning deaths in children under 6 years of age in the United States. The FDA has taken steps to prevent accidental iron poisoning of children by requiring warnings on iron supplements (FDA 1997).

Acute iron poisoning has little to do with the iron excess diseases associated with aging. These diseases result from long-term exposure to low-level excessive dietary iron.

Iron is a cumulative poison, and most of its toxic effects are seen as diseases of aging. Francesco S. Facchini, MD, referred very accurately to iron as "the aging factor" (Facchini 2002). Iron is a pro-oxidant and contributes to all aspects of aging.

How Much Dietary Iron Do Most Adults Need?

Men: The EAR (Estimated Average Requirement) for all men 19 years and older is 6 mg iron/day, and the RDA is 8 mg iron/day. The median intake is 16-18 mg iron/day.

Post-Menopausal Women: The EAR for iron for women over 51 years is 5 mg/day; the RDA is 8 mg/day. Median iron ingestion for these women is 12 mg/day.

	EAR	RDA	Median Intake
Men	6 mg/day	8 mg/day	16-18 mg/day
Post-Menopausal Women	5 mg/day	8 mg/day	12 mg/day

It is clear that a major portion of the U.S. population—those most susceptible to iron storage and toxic effects—are currently consuming much more iron than the amount necessary for healthy iron balance. Given the Panel on Micronutrients estimated that one half of the dietary iron comes from fortified foods, it seems apparent that if foods for adults were not fortified with iron, iron ingestion for the majority of people would be very close to the EAR and RDA.

Infant Iron Nutrition

Throughout history, most infants have been fed by mother's milk or by the milk of a nurse-maid. However, during the 1940s toward the end of the World War II, it became fashionable to bottle feed infants, and the first modified cow milk infant formulas emerged. Of course, iron was added as one of the modifications just to be certain these infants were getting enough iron. It was very quickly realized that bottle-fed infants are far more prone to microbial infection than are their breast-fed counterparts.

One reason for this was quickly realized: When an infant emerges from its mother's womb, the infant's immune system is undeveloped. Immune bodies are manufactured by each baby as that baby comes into contact with infectious organisms, there being no infectious organisms in the mother's womb. Nature has provided for this. Immunoglobins (IgG) entering from mother's milk are absorbed intact by the baby and, thereby, confer passive immunity on the infant. Three to six months after delivery, the baby's intestinal wall becomes a barrier, and intact proteins are no longer absorbed.

Passive immunity conferred on breast-fed infants is only one of the reasons for greater susceptibility of bottle-fed infants to microbial pathogens. Another important factor deals with antibiotic effects of iron withholding, but this factor was not initially recognized. Iron withholding as a defense against disease was first expressed in 1966 in an article by Eugene Weinberg entitled, "Roles of metallic ions in host-parasite interactions" (Weinberg 1966).

How Much Iron Does an Infant Need?

Before we discuss the iron withholding mechanism, we should examine an infant's need for dietary iron. Readers of this article will probably be surprised to learn that infants from 0 through 6 months need virtually no dietary iron. Here is the way the 2001 DRIs evaluate the adequate intake (AI) for iron for infants 0 through 6 months: "For this age group, it is assumed that the iron provided by human milk is adequate to meet the iron needs of the infant exclusively fed human milk from birth through 6 months. Therefore, the AI for young infants is based on the daily amount of iron secreted in human milk. The average iron concentration in human milk is 0.35 mg/L. Therefore the AI is set at 0.27 mg/day (0.78 L/day x 0.35 mg/L)." (Food and Nutrition Board 2001, pp 316-17.)

Of course, the people who established the adequate intake of iron for infants express their suspicion that nature may have made a mistake in providing so little iron in milk: "...there should be no expectation that an intake of 0.27 mg/day is adequate to meet the needs of almost all individual infants and, therefore, should be applied with extreme care." (Food and Nutrition Board 2001.) Because the American Academy of Pediatrics and the Canadian Pediatric Society recommend breast feeding for the first 6 months, the framers of the DRIs imply that the use of iron supplements may be necessary for exclusively breast-fed infants. Consequently, infant formula is supplemented with 1.8 mg iron per 100 calories. This amounts to 36mg per 2000 calories, or twice as much as the inflated DV for adults. We now examine the evidence that iron supplementation during early infancy is contrary to nature's intentions, and may actually promote growth of infectious organisms.

Iron Withholding as a Defense Strategy

Virtually all microorganisms require iron for reproduction and growth. There are some exceptions; in particular, some *Lactobacilli* and related non-pathogenic microbes actually live an iron-free existence. These human-friendly bacteria colonize an infant's intestinal tract soon after birth—more about these microbes later; it is the pathogenic, iron-dependent microbes that interest us here. Because these pathogens require iron, natural defense mechanisms have been developed to deprive them of iron, thereby preventing growth of the pathogens.

This part of the iron story begins with bird eggs. Why, given eggs are ordinarily laid in areas that are packed with bacteria and fungi, do bird embryos survive? The answer was discovered by Schade and Caroline (1944). The bird embryo develops in the yolk of the egg. All of the iron in an egg is concentrated in the yolk, which is completely encased by iron-free egg white. Schade and Caroline discovered that a certain fraction of the protein in egg white inhibits growth of pathogenic organisms, and that it does so by restricting the amount of iron available to the organism.

This fraction of egg white had been known for many years and was referred to as "ovalbumin." Schade and Caroline renamed ovalbumin, "siderophilin." ("Sidero" refers to iron, and "philin" refers to "the love of.") Thus, "siderophilin" is, by literal interpretation, an "iron-loving protein."

Later, Schade and Caroline (1946) isolated an iron-loving protein from blood serum. This protein also has powerful bacteriostatic properties. One important function of the serum-derived siderophile is to transport iron throughout the body. The serum-derived factor was designated "transferrin." ("Ferrin," like "sidero," refers to "iron.") Thus, transferrin is the protein that transports iron throughout the human body.

"Siderophilin" was renamed "ovotransferrin" to indicate a relationship with serum-derived transferrin. Thus, by 1946, two important antibiotic iron-binding proteins had been discovered: transferrin and ovotransferrin. We will discuss these proteins in greater detail, and will return to the interesting nomenclature for iron-binding compounds, in a later chapter.

However, first we must introduce two more characters that play important roles in iron metabolism in adults as well as infants: One is a siderophilic protein known as lactoferrin. The other is an enzyme known as xanthine oxidase.

Lactoferrin and Xanthine Oxidase

Biochemists go to great lengths in order to name enzymes according to their function. Xanthine is a breakdown product of nucleic acids. Xanthine oxidase, then, is an enzyme that oxidizes xanthine. When xanthine oxidase oxidises xanthine, a compound known as uric acid is produced. Some uric acid can be excreted in the urine. Uric acid is fairly insoluble so, if the amount of uric acid produced is in excess of the amount that can be excreted, crystals of uric acid can deposit in joints, resulting in a painful arthritic condition know as gout. We are not very interested in xanthine in this article, other than to note that xanthine and its oxidizing enzyme are present in milk. Xanthine and xanthine oxidase are also found in all cells of the body.

Xanthine oxidase is a very complex enzyme that contains riboflavin (vitamin B_2), molybdenum, and iron. Here we find another function of xanthine oxidase. Xanthine oxidase also oxidizes iron (Topham et al. 1982). The iron bound to the active site of the enzyme is in the iron II (ferrous iron) oxidation state. When iron is oxidized to iron III (ferric iron), it is released from the enzyme.

Lactoferrin refers to an iron-binding protein found in milk. Colostrum is the richest source of lactoferrin, followed by milk.

However, the name doesn't really do lactoferrin justice because lactoferrin is not limited to milk. Lactoferrin is found in many body secretions: lachrymal glands (tear glands), mammary glands, and secretions of respiratory, gastrointestinal, and genital tracts. Lactoferrin binds iron very tightly—about 240 times as tightly as does transferrin. By binding iron so tightly, lactoferrin deprives microbes of iron, and it is considered the first line of defense against microbial infection. (Weinberg 2005)

Lactoferrin, abundant in milk, binds only iron (III). Thus, as soon as iron III is released from xanthine oxidase, lactoferrin binds the iron, thereby maintaining a virtually iron-free infant intestinal system. This is critical as most pathogens cannot grow in this environment—only certain *Lactobacilli* and related nonpathogenic organisms can grow in the absence of iron.

The lactoferrin/xanthine oxidase relationship is therefore the most important factor preventing growth of pathogens while ensuring that non-pathogenic bacteria colonize the previously sterile intestines of the newborn. Addition of iron to an infant diet, therefore, can have serious consequences.

Sweden Terminated Iron Fortification

Following the lead of the U.S. and Canada, Sweden joined ranks and initiated an iron-fortification program in the 1950s. People from Sweden and Finland have a high incidence of hereditary hemochromatosis. The National Food Administration of Sweden determined that the evidence that iron fortification of food was harming this target group was significant enough to terminate the program. The iron fortification of food in Sweden was withdrawn on January 1, 1995 (Olsson et al. 1997).

It is interesting that no mention is made of the Swedish experience in the 2001 DRIs. Why? It is very likely that not one of the 14 members of the Panel on Micronutrients was even aware of actions of the Swedish National Food Administration. The U.S. Food and Nutrition Board and Health Canada should carefully follow the results of the Swedish experiment!

REFERENCES

Facchini FS. 2002. *The Iron Factor of Aging*, Tucson, AZ: Fenestra Books.

FDA. 1997. Iron-Containing Supplements and Drugs: Label Warning Statements and Unit-Dose Packaging Requirements. Federal Register 62 FR 2217.

Food and Nutrition Board, Institute of Medicine. 1993. *Iron Deficiency Anemia: Recommended Guidelines for the Prevention, Detection, and Management Among U.S. Children and Women of Childbearing Age.* Washington: National Academy Press.

———— 2001. *Dietary Reference Intakes for Vitamin A, Vitamin K, Arsenic, Boron, Chromium, Copper, Iodine, Iron, Manganese, Molybdenum, Nickel, Silicon, Vanadium, and Zinc.* Washington: National Academy Press.

Gura T. 1999. New genes boost rice nutrients. Science. 285:994-5.

Lee DH, Jacobs DR Jr. 2005 Interaction among heme iron, zinc, and supplemental vitamin C intake on the risk of lung cancer: Iowa Women's Health Study. Nutr Cancer 52(2):130-7.

Murray MJ, Murray AB, Murray MB, Murray CJ. 1978. The adverse effect of iron repletion on the course of certain infections. Br Med J. 2:1113.

Olsson KS, Väisänen M, Konar J, Bruce Å. 1997. The effect of withdrawal of food iron fortification in Sweden as studied with phlebotomy in subjects with genetic hemochromatosis. EJCN. 51(11):782-6.

Shade AL, Caroline L. 1944. Raw hen egg white and the role of iron in growth inhibition of *Shigella dysenteria, Staphylococcus aureus, Escherichia coli,* and *Saccharomyces cerevisiae.* Science. 100:14-15.

———— 1946. An iron-binding component in human blood plasma. Science. 104:340-41.

Tappel A. 2007. Heme of consumed red meat can act as a catalyst of oxidative damage and could initiate colon, breast and prostate cancers, heart disease and other diseases. Med Hypothesis. 68(3):562-4.

Topham RW, Walker MC, Callisch MP, Williams RW. 1982. Evidence for the participation of intestinal xanthine oxidase in the mucosal processing of iron. Biochemistry. 21:4529.

Weinberg ED. 1966. Roles of metallic ions in host-parasite interactions. Bacteriological Reviews. 30:1336-51.

———— 1974. Iron and susceptibility to infectious disease. Science. 184:952-56.

———— 2005. Iron withholding as a defense strategy. In: Weiss G, Gordeuk VR, Hershko C, eds. *Anemia of Chronic Disease*. Boca Raton: Taylor & Francis.

Whittaker P, Dunkel VC, Seifried HE, Clarke JJ, San RHC. 2002. Evaluation of iron chelators for assessing the mechanism of genotoxicity of iron compounds. FDA Science Forum Poster Abstract, Board Z-06.

Whittaker P, Tufaro PR, Dunkel VC, Rader JI. 2001. Fortification of iron and folate in Cereals. FDA Science Forum Poster Abstract, Board P02.

Chapter 4

Maintaining Body Iron Balance

Iron Distribution in Humans

The total amount of iron in an adult woman is around 2-3 g (~45 mg/kg) while that in a man is around 3.5-5 g (~55 mg/kg). Approximately 60-70% of the body's iron is found circulating in the blood, tightly bound within the heme matrix of hemoglobin. When bound within heme, iron is maintained in the divalent state [iron (II)]. The function of heme-bound iron is to carry oxygen to all cells for cellular metabolism. Once hemoglobin has released its oxygen to a cell, it then transports carbon dioxide away from these cells. Although the carbon dioxide is not bound to the iron, the intact hemoglobin molecule is responsible for transporting around 15% of the carbon dioxide released by catabolism. Thus, iron [iron (II)] is important both for delivering oxygen to cells and for removing carbon dioxide from cells.

The second most abundant supply of iron is stored in the liver cells and endothelial macrophages, within a cave-like structure known as ferritin. Each ferritin 'cage' can hold up to 4500 atoms of trivalent iron [iron(III)]. This storage iron can be released when the body needs it. Approximately 20-30% of the body's iron resides within ferritin 'cages.' When iron breaks out of its cage, hemosiderin—a breakdown product of ferritin—is released. Under healthy circumstances, some hemosiderin-bound iron is present in the liver and other body tissues.

A small amount (~3 mg) of trivalent iron [iron(III)] is attached to transferrin—the iron-transport glycoprotein. Iron(III) is virtually insoluble at physiologic pH. However, transferrin binding allows iron(III) to be soluble in the blood plasma. Each molecule of transferrin can carry two atoms of iron(III). Iron(III) is very tightly bound to transferrin, preventing redox cycling of the iron. Even though a very small amount of iron is transferrin-bound, this iron is of unusual clinical significance. Under healthy circumstances, transferrin is around 30-35% saturated with iron.

The remaining body iron is localized in myoglobin—iron-containing enzymes—and within mitochondria in cytochromes and iron-sulfur clusters. Myoglobin iron is found in muscle and provides a source of iron for muscle metabolism. Within mitochondria, iron functions to transfer electrons in the electron transport chain, which generates energy that is captured in the form of high-energy phosphate bonds (ATP).

When heme bonds are ruptured, the iron is oxidized to its trivalent state [iron(III)], and is rapidly bound to transferrin and recycled. If erythrocyte heme levels are adequate, some of the iron released

Table 3: Distribution of iron in a 70-kg adult male.[1]
Data taken from Papanikolaou and Pantopoulos, 2005.

Hemoglobin in red blood cells	~1800 mg
Iron stores (liver ferritin and hemosiderin)	~1000 mg
Endothelial macrophages	~600 mg
Muscle (myoglobin)	~300 mg
Bone marrow	~300 mg
Plasma transferrin	~3 mg
[1]In an adult female of similar weight, the amount of storage iron generally would be less.	

from heme will go to storage in the liver or in macrophages in the reticuloendothelial system.

When iron storage gets excessive, ferritin is degraded to hemosiderin. Release of hemosiderin gives rise to the term, "hemosiderosis," for the condition found among the South Africans consuming excessive iron.

There is No Physiological Mechanism for Iron Excretion

Perhaps the single most important factor resulting in iron's toxicity is the fact that humans do not possess any physiological pathway for excretion of iron. A healthy individual absorbs around 1-2 mg iron each day and loses approximately the same amount. Iron is lost by nonspecific methods that involve desquamation of skin cells and intestinal cells, but no active excretory mechanism exists. This feature of iron physiology has been known for many years. It was first reported in 1979 by the great iron expert, T.H. Bothwell (Bothwell et al. 1979).

Consider the implications of this strange quirk of nature in view of the Estimated Adult Requirement (EAR) for iron set by the 2001 DRIs (Food and Nutrition Board 2001), and the excessive amounts of iron that we are consuming in iron-adulterated foods. The EAR for men was established by a valid method of factorial modeling that took into consideration basal iron losses and weight. Using this method, with data from 13 iron balance studies, the EAR for men is set at 6 mg/day.

The Recommended Dietary Intake (RDA) was set by modeling the components of iron requirements and estimating the requirement for absorbed iron at the ninety-seven and one-half percentile. An upper limit of 18 percent iron absorption was used to establish the RDA, which is 8 mg/day for men.

Again, the 2001 DRIs state that the median dietary intake of iron is approximately 16 to 18 mg. This is two times the RDA. More than one-half of this intake is being delivered in foods to which iron has been added, i.e., iron-adulterated foods.

Females of Childbearing Age

Women have greater iron losses and absorb a greater percentage of iron from food than do men. The Food and Nutrition Board (1993, p 43-44) summarizes the situation for women:

> Average menstrual blood loss is about 30 ml/month, but 10 percent of women regularly lose more than 80 ml/month and are likely to become anemic because their iron loss is usually greater than that which can be compensated for by increased absorption of iron from the diet.... Menstrual blood loss varies with some methods of contraception, roughly decreasing to half with oral contraceptives and doubling with intrauterine devices (IUDs).... Pregnancy imposes increased iron needs for the growth of the fetus and for expansion of maternal blood volume. Even women who are not iron deficient at the beginning of a pregnancy...are at risk of developing an iron-responsive depression in hemoglobin concentrations in the third trimester unless they receive supplemental iron.

Iron Absorption and Storage

Because there is no physiologic mechanism for actively excreting iron, body iron homeostasis is maintained primarily by a complex interaction of a variety of factors, both dietary and internal. The most significant factors involve iron absorption and storage:

1. Controlling iron absorption.
   a. Type of dietary iron:
      i. Heme iron: Very absorbable (~30-40%)
      ii. Iron ascorbate: Very absorbable (~30-40%)
      iii. Iron salts: Absorb ~8-15%.
      iv. "Free" iron (Fe^0): As iron carbonyl, less absorbable than iron salts.
      v. Phosphorous and phytate—iron absorption blockers.
   b. Mucosal block: Ingestion of a large amount of iron in a single dose causes absorptive intestinal cells to resist

iron absorption for several days.
  c. Ferritin stores regulation: In iron-deficient conditions, iron absorption is significantly stimulated, by two- or threefold.
  d. Erythropoietic regulation: Hepcidin (see below).
  2. Iron storage within ferritin, in liver cells and macrophages— adequate ferritin iron stores inhibit iron absorption.

Hepcidin

"Each day, almost 200 billion red blood cells are produced in the normal adult to replace a like number reaching the end of their life span. Each red cell contains more than a billion atoms of iron, four in each tetrameric molecule of haemoglobin, so that more than 200 quintillion (200 x 10^{18}) atoms of iron are needed daily for erythropoiesis or almost 20 mg of iron by weight. Human iron metabolism is distinguished by an efficient cycling of iron from recently destroyed to newly formed red cells. Normally, less than 0.05% of the total body iron is acquired or lost each day, making humans unique among animals in the effectiveness with which iron is conserved." (Brittenham 1994)

Erythropoiesis refers to the synthesis of red blood cells (erythrocytes). This process takes place in bone marrow. Erythropoiesis requires approximately 25-30 mg of iron/day. This iron comes primarily from recycling of iron via reticuloendothelial macrophages that ingest senescent red blood cells. Approximately 20 mL of red blood cells are catabolized per day, releasing approximately 25-30 mg iron, which is recycled.

When additional iron is required for erythropoiesis, a signal is transmitted from bone marrow to the liver, and the liver responds by inhibiting synthesis of a polypeptide known as hepcidin. Hepcidin inhibits iron absorption by binding to and inactivating ferroportin. Thus, preventing hepcidin synthesis—the signal from bone marrow that more iron is required for erythropoiesis—causes the necessary increased absorption. The signal from bone marrow to the liver is being actively investigated, but is still not known.

Hepcidin was initially isolated from ultrafiltrates of plasma and urine (Krause et al. 2000). Hepcidin is one of many polypeptides found in blood and urine that have antimicrobial properties. In contrast to other antimicrobial peptides, hepcidin is predominantly expressed in the liver (Parks et al. 2001). Under physiological conditions, humans produce and maintain relatively stable levels of hepcidin. Low hepcidin levels trigger increased iron absorption from the duodenum and iron release from reticuloendothelial macrophages. Similarly, when iron stores are satisfied, hepcidin expression increases causing a decrease in iron absorption from the duodenum, and iron release from reticuloendothelial macrophages (Papanikolaou and Pantopoulos 2005).

Transferrin and Transferrin Receptors

Iron is transported in blood plasma attached to a glycoprotein that is synthesized in the liver. The glycoprotein is appropriately known as transferrin (Tf). Each transferrin molecule can carry 2 atoms of Fe(III). The iron is tightly bound to its glycoprotein carrier, which prevents it from redox cycling. In healthy individuals, transferrin is around 30-35% saturated. Higher levels of transferrin loading indicate iron excess; low levels of transferrin loading indicate iron deficit. Transferrin loading is one of the most important measures of iron status of an individual.

Receptors for iron-loaded transferrin are found on the surface of every cell. Some cells have thousands of transferrin receptors. The larger the number of transferrin receptors, the greater the capacity for iron uptake. The most carefully studied transferrin receptor is referred to as TfR1 (transferrin receptor 1). When the iron-loaded transferrin attaches to the transferrin receptor, the transferrin-transferrin receptor complex is endocytosed (transported into the cell while encapsulated in a structure known as an endosome). The endosome concentrates hydrogen ions from the cellular milieu, causing the pH of the endosome to lower.

The lowered pH results in release of the iron from transferrin, as divalent iron [Fe(II)]. Once transferrin has released its iron load, the apotransferrin (the ironless glycoprotein) is recycled. When the iron(II) is released from transferrin, it is picked up by another protein, known as the divalent metal transporter. The divalent metal transporter then transports the iron across the endosomal membrane. The internalized iron is incorporated into iron-containing proteins, and the excess is detoxified by sequestration into ferritin (Brock et al. 1994).

The divalent metal transporter is a non-specific transport protein so it also carries other divalent metal ions such as zinc(II), manganese(II), and copper(II). This poses a problem for people who ingest too much iron because iron(II) competes with zinc(II), so excess dietary iron may precipitate zinc deficiency in a person with marginal zinc intake. Refer to the 2001 DRIs for a discussion of iron-zinc interactions (Food and Nutrition Board 2001, pp 357-58).

Once iron has entered a cell, it must be transported to organelles such as mitochondria. Very little is known about this aspect of iron transport, but it is presumed that the iron is chelated by small molecules such as citrate, ascorbate, or polyphosphates.

Lactoferrin

Transferrin is the iron-binding and transporting glycoprotein found in plasma, lymph, and cerebrospinal fluid. Transferrin-binding maintains iron in the iron(III) oxidation state, and effectively prevents iron from redox cycling in plasma, lymph, and cerebrospinal fluid.

Lactoferrin is also an iron(III)-binding glycoprotein. Lactoferrin is found in secretions of lachrymal glands (tear ducts), mammary glands, and of respiratory, gastrointestinal, and genital tracts. These are the major sites for entrance of microbial pathogens. Similar to transferrin, each lactoferrin molecule can bind 2 atoms of iron(III). Lactoferrin binds iron(III) about 240 times as efficiently as does transferrin. As well, lactoferrin continues to bind iron(III) even at low pH values. This very tight binding is the basis for antibiotic properties of lactoferrin.

Virtually all pathogenic microorganisms require iron for reproduction. A few non-pathogenic microbes are known to live an iron-free existence—*Lactobacilli* and some related human-friendly microbes that colonize the intestinal tract shortly after birth. One pathogenic microorganism (*Borrelia burgdorferi,* the cause of Lyme disease) has been found to survive in the absence of iron (Posey and Gheradini 2000). These bacteria employ manganese and cobalt as mineral catalysts.

Lactoferrin, along with other antibiotic factors such as lysozyme, constitute the first line of defense against infection. Lactoferrin prevents reproduction of pathogens while lysozyme destroys these organisms by cutting holes in the biomembrane that surrounds and protects the microbes.

Iron withholding as a defense against infection was first suggested by Eugene Weinberg in 1966 (Weinberg 1966). By 1987, many studies had demonstrated the validity of this suggestion, and an entire book appeared on the subject (Bullen and Griffiths 1987). Currently, iron withholding as a preventive against infection is a fundamental concept in the clinical chemistry of infection. Recombinant bovine and human lactoferrin are now available for studies on nutraceutical/ preservative/pharmaceutical properties (Weinberg 2007).

Regulation of Cellular Iron Metabolism

We have examined over-all iron homeostasis and physiology but have not discussed the details regarding how cells handle iron. This is an exciting field; however, it is currently under construction. Cellular iron metabolism is regulated by interaction of iron responsive elements (IREs) and iron regulatory proteins (IRPs). We won't go into the details in this article. For the interested reader, the known details of cellular iron regulation have been summarized recently (Papanikolaou and Pantopoulos 2005).

How Can You Determine Your Iron Status?

Many women take iron supplements regularly. However, it should be clear by now that iron supplementation should be approached with great caution. Iron supplements should **not** be taken simply due to periodic feelings of weakness and lethargy that occurs during periodic loss of blood. Only assessment of the body's iron status can indicate whether an iron-containing supplement should be taken.

This assessment might include: red cell count, blood hemoglobin, mean corpuscular volume, hematocrit, mean corpuscular hemoglobin (pg/red cell), mean corpuscular hemoglobin concentration (g/dc RBC), transferrin loading, and serum ferritin.

The most important measurements are: 1) transferrin-bound iron; 2) total iron binding capacity (TIBC); 3) transferrin saturation; 4) serum ferritin. Table 4 gives normal values for these measurements.

Table 4. Normal Values for Transferrin-bound Iron, Total Iron Binding Capacity (TIBC), and Transferrin Saturation[a]

Measurement	
Transferrin iron	**60-170 mcg/dl[b]**
TIBC	**240-450 mcg/dl[b]**
Transferrin saturation	**25-35%**
Serum Ferritin	**25-75 ng/ml[c]**

[a]Normal values may vary from laboratory to laboratory
[b]Micrograms per deciliter
[c]Nanograms per milliliter

According to the Food and Nutrition Board (1993), having low values for two of these three measures indicates anemia. Similarly, although the Food and Nutrition Board doesn't state it, having elevated levels of any two of these three values contraindicates use of an iron supplement.

What To Do For Abnormal Blood Iron

Low Blood Values: As indicated by the Food and Nutrition Board (1993), low blood values for two of the primary measurements may indicate iron-deficiency anemia. True iron deficiency anemia is reversed by taking an iron supplement, which should be supervised by a physician, and continued only as long as is necessary for the blood parameters to return to normal values.

Elevated Blood Values:
1. Elevated transferrin iron, TIBC, transferrin saturation, and/or serum ferritin likely indicates an iron overloaded system.
2. If blood parameters indicate iron overload, it would be wise to be genetically tested for hereditary hemochromatosis.
3. If you have hereditary hemochromatosis, seek medical attention immediately.

Methods for reducing elevated iron levels:
1. Donate blood: This is the most readily accessible method, and results are better than with any other method.
2. Prevent iron absorption.
   a. Avoid heme iron.
   b. Avoid all iron-containing supplements.
   c. Eat foods high in phytate (legumes, brown rice, and other minimally refined grains that have not been adulterated by the addition of iron). Phytate and other forms of organic phosphorous bind iron in the intestine and prevent its absorption.
   d. Rice bran is a rich source of phytate. Phytate is also referred to as inositol hexaphosphate (IP6). An extract of rice bran, high in IP6, is marketed by Tsuno Foods & Rice Company, Wakayama, Japan (Sardi 1999).
   e. Because iron is a pro-oxidant, antioxidants may help protect from some of the damaging effects of excess iron. A later

chapter of this book will discuss the roles of antioxidants in detail. Antioxidants do not result in reduced body iron stores.

3. Chelation therapy: Ordinarily, chelation therapy should be reserved for those with severe iron overload, such as occurs in transfusion siderosis. A modified deferrioxamine that can be taken orally is a specific and powerful iron-chelator. Exjade® (deferasirox), manufactured by Novartis Pharmaceutical Corporation in Stein, Switzerland, was FDA approved in 2005, for use in transfusion siderosis.

A Note on Zeolite

Don't be too zealous about zeolite! Zeolites are aluminosilicate members of microporous solids known as molecular sieves. More than 150 zeolite types have been synthesized, and 48 naturally occurring zeolites are known. Natural zeolites form where volcanic rocks and ash layers react with alkaline groundwater, and are also found crystallized in shallow marine environments. The world's annual production of natural zeolite is around 4 million tons. More than half of the mined zeolite is shipped to China where it is used in the concrete industry.

Zeolites have an open structure that can accommodate a wide variety of cations, such as Na^+, K^+, Ca^{2+}, Mg^{2+}, Zn^{2+}, Mn^{2+}, Cu^{2+}, and are currently marketed by companies that claim they can remove heavy metals from the human body. This claim is not true. Zeolites may bind metals and prevent their absorption, but zeolites have no ability to remove heavy metals (or iron) from the human body. Overuse of zeolites will likely prevent absorption of essential nutrients such as magnesium, calcium, and zinc, but will not bring about the removal of toxic metals.

REFERENCES

Bothwell TH, Charlton AW, Cook JD, Finch CA. 1979. Iron Metabolism in Man. Blackwell Scientific Publications, Oxford.

Brittenham GM. 1994. The red cell cycle. In Brock JH, Halliday JW,

Pippard MG, Powell LW. 1994. *Iron Metabolism in Health and Disease.* London, Philadelphia, Toronto, Sydney, Tokyo: W.B. Saunders Company Ltd.

Brock JH, Halliday JW, Pippard MG, Powell LW. 1994. *Iron Metabolism in Health and Disease.* London, Philadelphia, Toronto, Sydney, Tokyo: W.B. Saunders Company Ltd.

Bullen JJ, Griffiths E. 1987. *Iron and Infection. Molecular, Physiological and Clinical Aspects.* Chichester, New York, Brisbane, Toronto, Singapore: John Wiley and Sons.

Food and Nutrition Board. 1993. *Iron Deficiency Anemia: Recommended Guidelines for the Prevention, Detection, and Management Among U.S. Children and Women of Childbearing Age.* Washington, DC: National Academy Press.

Krause A, Neitz S, Magert HJ, Schulz A, Forssmann WG, Schula A, Forssmann WG, Schulz-Knappe P, Adermann K. 2000. LEAP-1, a novel highly disulfide-bonded human peptide, exhibits antimicrobial activity. FEBS Lett. 480:147-50.

Papanikolaou G, Pantopoulos K. 2005. Iron metabolism and toxicity. Toxicology and Applied Pharmacology. 202:199-211.

Park CH, Valore EV, Waring AJ, Ganz T. 2001. Hepcidin, a urinary antimicrobial peptide synthesized in the liver. J Biol Chem. 278(11):7806-816.

Posey JE, Gherardini FC. 2000. Lack of a role for iron in the Lyme disease pathogen. Science. 288:1651.

Sardi B. 1999. *The Iron Time Bomb.* San Dimas, CA: Bill Sardi.

Weinberg ED. 1966. Roles of metallic ions in host-parasite interactions. Bact Reviews. 30:1336-51.

———— 2007. Antibiotic properties and applications of lactoferrin. Cur Pharm Design. 13:801-811.

Chapter 5

The 2001 DRIs: Iron
Hazard Identification

Pitifully Inadequate

The Food and Nutrition Board, Institute of Medicine, is responsible for setting the Recommended Dietary Allowances (RDAs), and presents its findings in a publication entitled, *Dietary Reference Intakes* (DRIs). This publication has a profound influence on nutrition-related practices for all North Americans. We rely on it in our daily lives, and have the right to expect that every effort has been made to establish valid guidelines that will benefit our health. Unfortunately, in the case of iron, the Board has failed to meet its obligation, and countless millions of people are at higher risk for several debilitating and fatal conditions.

The RDAs for iron were established using valid methods—there is no reason to question the RDAs for iron. However, we might ask why, when the RDA for iron was set at 8 mg/day for all adults other than women of childbearing age, and when the Board indicated that this group is consuming an estimated 18 mg/day, did they not call attention to this fact? The Board indicated that more than half of the iron that is being consumed comes from foods to which iron is added. It should have been apparent to the Board that if foods were not adulterated by the addition of iron, the iron intake would be very close to the RDA. Their actions are unacceptable. In this chapter, we will review the section on "Iron Hazard Identification" presented in the 2001 DRIs, and identify areas of iron toxicity that were not included.

The section on "Iron Hazard Identification" in the 2001 DRIs is pitifully inadequate and constitutes an assault on the health of the entire North American population. This section makes no mention of iron's neurotoxicity. Nor does it mention the role of iron in arthritis, adult onset diabetes, hypogonadism and impotency, ocular degeneration, osteoporosis, and other diseases of aging. We will now examine the 2001 DRIs review of iron toxicology in some detail. Subsequent chapters will deal with the information that was not included in that review.

The Debate

The debate over iron adulteration of food was initiated in 1970-1971 when the FDA put forth a recommendation to triple the amount of iron added to food. As stated previously, the Commissioner of the FDA examined the evidence and concluded that there should be no increase. However, in spite of the Commissioner's recommendations, a 50% increase was mandated.

The debate reached a point of culmination in 1986 with the publication of two articles in *Nutrition Today.*

1. One of these articles was by John L Beard, Department of Nutrition, Pennsylvania University. The title is, "Iron fortification – rationale and effects." (*Nutrition Today*, July/August 1986, 17-20.) Dr. Beard argued that the food fortification had been effective, but could be made more effective by increasing the amount of iron that is added to food.

2. William Crosby, Director of Hematology at the Chapman Cancer Center in Joplin Missouri wrote the rebuttal article, "Yin, yang and iron." (*Nutrition Today*, July/August 1986, 14-16.) Dr. Crosby argued that iron is carcinogenic and should not be added to the human food supply.

In the intervening years from 1986 to 2001 when the DRIs

were published, iron's toxicity to the nervous system became firmly established. Yet there is not a single reference to iron as a neurotoxin in the iron toxicology section of the DRIs. Why?

The Panel on Micronutrients

The Panel on Micronutrients of the U.S. Food and Nutrition Board is responsible for the section on iron in the 2001 DRIs. The panel consisted of fourteen members and two consultants. Not one of these members or consultants was versed in iron toxicology. However, it was necessary to select someone to write this section. John Beard, who favored increasing the level of iron added to food, was selected to write the section on "Iron Hazard Identification."

Iron Hazard Identification

The section on Hazard Identification for iron is divided into the following subsections:

- **Introductory**. Presentation of redox cycling and oxygen radical generation by iron.
- **Acute Effects**. "There are reports of acute toxicity resulting from overdoses of medicinal iron, especially in young children. Accidental iron over-dose is the most common cause of poisoning deaths in children under 6 years of age in the United States."
- **Iron-Zinc Interactions**. "High intakes of iron supplements have been associated with reduced zinc absorption as measured by changes in serum zinc concentrations after dosing."
- **Gastrointestinal Effects**. "High-dose iron supplements are commonly associated with constipation and other gastrointestinal effects including nausea, vomiting, and diarrhea."
- **Secondary Iron Overload.** "Secondary iron overload occurs when the body iron stores are increased as a consequence of parenteral iron administration, repeated

blood transfusions, or hematological disorders that increase the rate of iron absorption."

- **Cardiovascular Disease.** The concluding paragraph in this section states, "Taken as a whole, this body of evidence does not provide convincing support for a causal relationship between the level of dietary iron intake and the risk for CHD (coronary heart disease). However, it is important to note that the evidence is insufficient to definitively exclude iron as a risk factor." (Unfortunately, Dr Beard is inaccurate when he states, "Taken as a whole..." because he did not cover the whole. A more comprehensive review will be found in chapter 7 dealing with Iron and Cardiovascular Diseases.)
- **Cancer.** "There is no doubt that iron accumulation in the liver is a risk factor for hepatocellular carcinoma in patients with hemochromatosis. However, the evidence for a relationship between dietary iron intake and cancer, particularly colon cancer, in the general population is inconclusive."
- **Identification of Distinct and Highly Sensitive Subpopulations.** This section contains a limited attempt to address the problem of iron accumulation in humans with hereditary hemochromatosis or related conditions. Like all other sections, Dr Beard's presentation of hereditary hemochromatosis is completely inadequate.

Missing Information

The section on Hazard Identification in the 2001 DRIs is incomplete in its discussions of iron in relation to heart disease and cancer—we will examine this later. As well, there was no mention of the role of iron in other pathologies. A list of the areas that were omitted includes:

- **Iron and Neurological Degeneration:**
  - **Parkinson's Disease**

- o Alzheimer's Disease
- o Huntington's Disease
- o Multiple Sclerosis and Other Demyelinating Diseases
- Iron and Infection
- Iron and the Endocrine Glands
  - o Adult-onset Diabetes
  - o Pituitary Malfunction
  - o Hypogonadism and Infertility
- Iron and Arthritis
- Iron and Osteoporosis
- Iron and Ocular Pathology—We cannot fault the 2001 DRIs, however, for failing to include a section on ocular pathology because most of this research has been elucidated since the 2001 DRIs were formulated.
- Iron and Other Diseases of Aging

In the next section, we will discuss the information omitted from the 2001 DRIs in regard to the most glaring omission: The neurotoxicity of iron.

Why Did the 2001 DRIs Not Discuss Iron Neurotoxicity

Oxidative metabolism in the brain is higher than in any other organ, so it is not surprising that the brain has higher levels of iron than any organ other than the liver. Brain iron homeostasis is crucial to health. Any disruption of brain or nerve tissue iron homeostasis is bound to result in damage.

The presence of iron in neurofibrillary tangles, senile plaques, and walls of the vasculature in Alzheimer's disease was first discussed in 1953 (Goodman 1953). Evidence of iron accumulation in the substantia nigra of people with Parkinson's disease started to accumulate in 1966, with a publication in Spanish, "Iron in the blood, cerebrospinal fluid and urine in patients with Parkinson's disease and in patients without this disorder." (Vecchiola et al. 1966.) In 1968, increased levels of iron in brain areas associated with epilepsy were reported (Rojas and Messen, 1968). Hence, by 1970, suspicion was developing that a number of neurodegenerative diseases might be linked to iron misregulation.

During the 1980s and '90s, these findings were confirmed and extended – many studies found increased iron in the substantia nigra of patients with Parkinson's disease and in the neurofibrillary tangles and senile plaques found in Alzheimer's disease. As well, iron accumulates in brain regions and nerve tissue associated with epilepsy, Huntington's disease, Hallervorden-Spatz disease, multiple sclerosis, and other demyelinating diseases. Brain and nerve tissue iron accumulation is now recognized as a cardinal feature of most, if not all, neurodegenerative diseases.

However, the 2001 DRIs made no statement regarding the neurotoxicity of iron. That is unfortunate because it was apparent long before 2001 that iron accumulates in brain regions and nerve tissue associated with most neurodegenerative diseases. The following references all appeared in ample time to be included in the toxicology section of the 2001 DRIs:

- **Alzheimer's disease**: Goodman 1953; Thompson et al. 1988; Blass and Gibson 1991; Connor et al. 1991; Connor et al. 1992; Connor et al. 1992; Connor 1992; Jellinger et al. 1990; Griffiths and Crossman 1993; Loeffler et al. 1995.
- **Parkinson's disease**: Vecchiola et al. 1966; Youdim et al. 1980; Cohen 1984; Langston 1988; Sofic et al. 1988; Dexter et al. 1989; Jenner 1989; Riedered et al. 1989; Youdim et al. 1989; Gotz et al. 1990; Jellinger et al. 1990; Ben-Shachar et al. 1990, 1991; Youdim et al. 1990; Carlsson and Fornstedt 1991; Dexter et al. 1991; Jenner 1991; Sofic et al. 1991; Youdim et al. 1991; Jenner 1992; Ben-Shachar et al. 1992; Olanow 1992; Olanow et al. 1992; Good et al. 1992; Jellinger et al. 1992; Jenner et al. 1992; Riederer and Lange 1992; Sengstock et al. 1992; Griffiths and Crossman 1993; Jenner 1993; Hirsch 1993; Nakano 1993; Yodim and Riederer 1993; Morris and Edwards 1994; Hirsch 1994; Enochs et al. 1994; Kienzl et al. 1995;

Mann et al. 1995;Montgomery Jr 1995; Nielsen et al. 1995;
Jenner and Olanow 1996; Ebadu et al. 1996; Owen et al.
1996; Galazka-Friedman and Friedman 1997; Jenner 1998;
Double et al. 1999; Jellinger 1999; Kienzl et al. 1999.
• **Huntington's and Hallervorden-Spatz disease**: Drayer et
al. 1987; Swaiman 1991; Bartzokis et al. 1999.
• **Multiple sclerosis and other demyelinating diseases**:
Esiri et al. 1976; Craelius et al. 1982; Valk 1989; Gocht and
Lohler 1990; Swaiman 1991.
• **Epilepsy**: Rojas and Messen 1968; Hughes and Oppenheimer
1969; Campbell et al. 1984; Jones and Hedley 1983; Ikeda
2001.
• **Psychiatric illnesses**: Jones and Hedley 1983; Cutler
1994.
• **Animal models** of neurodegenerative diseases: Ben-
Shachar and Youdim 1991; Tanaka 1991; Temlett et al.
1994; Hall et al. 1992; Smith et al. 1998; Han et al. 1999;
Berg et al. 1999; Yantin and Anderson 1999.

Clearly, when the 2001 DRIs were being formulated, there was
ample evidence that iron causes oxidative damage that either initiates
or contributes to the progress of each of these diseased conditions.

Examples of Iron Accumulation in Neurodegenerative Diseases

The references listed below demonstrate elevated iron levels in
brain regions associated with various neurological diseases. Some
representative examples given here indicate the nature of these
findings. Sofic et al (1988) described the postmortem brain iron
content of individuals who had Parkinson's disease and demonstrated
a 176% increase in total iron, and a 255% increase in ferric iron
in the substantia nigra; no changes were observed in the cortex,
hippocampus, putamen, or globus pallidus. Iron deposits are found in
the plaques surrounding nerves found in multiple sclerosis (Craelium
et al. 1982), and in senile plaques in Alzheimer's disease (Connor et

al. 1991; Connor 1992; Connor et al. 1992; Thompson et al. 1988).

High Iron Levels and Neurodegeneration

It is still uncertain whether excess iron in the substantia nigra is a cause of Parkinson's, or if it is a secondary factor that accelerates nerve damage. Similarly, the role of iron in the neurofibrillary tangles in Alzheimer's disease and in nodules surrounding demyelating nerves is still unclear. It is likely that both pathways make a contribution.

Shoham and Youdim (2004) have demonstrated that nutritional iron deprivation can alleviate chemically-induced neurodegeneration in rats. A recent article demonstrates that iron overload can initiate neurological degeneration in laboratory animals (Jiang et al. 2007). Injecting rats with iron dextran resulted in iron accumulation in dopaminergic neurons associated with Parkinson's disease. This accumulated iron resulted in a decrease in dopamine content of these nerves, and decreased their ability to secrete dopamine. These studies indicate that chronic iron overload can cause neurodegeneration, and nutritional iron restriction can help prevent some neurodegenerative conditions.

One way or the other, the iron is present in brain and nerve tissue in humans afflicted by these diseases, and its removal is a major thrust in the treatment of many neurodegenerative diseases.

Iron Chelation Therapy

Several new drugs that incorporate both an iron chelator and an antioxidant (monoamine oxidase inhibitor) have been developed to treat Parkinson's and Alzheimer's patients (Youdim et al. 2004, 2005; Amit et al. 2007). The purpose of the chelator is to remove iron; the monoamine oxidase inhibitor is intended to prevent damage caused by oxidation of dopamine, which produces the powerful neurotoxin, 6-hydroxydopamine. It would be far better to prevent the iron from accumulating, and one way might be to stop iron adulteration of food.

Conclusions

The references for this chapter speak for themselves. References are arranged in historical sequence, from 1955 to 2007. Every study listed here confirms high iron levels in specific brain regions and nerve tissue associated with each type of neurodegenerative disease. I have not been able to find any contradictory information in the published medical literature—every study that has examined iron levels in neurons associated with each respective disease has found increased levels when compared to normal brains.

By the time Dr. Beard was writing the section on Iron Hazard Identification for the 2001 DRIs, more than 100 published papers clearly documented the accumulation of iron in neurodegenerative diseases. How could anyone overlook this information? Dr. Beard overlooked it, as did the fourteen members and two consultants of the Panel on Micronutrients, all of whom accepted Dr. Beard's completely unacceptable review.

REFERENCES

1955-1979

Esiri MM, Taylor CR, Mason DY. 1976. Applications of an immuno-peroxidase method to a study of the central nervous system: Preliminary findings in a study of human formalin-fixed material. Neuropathol Appl Neurobiol. 2:233-46.

Goodman L. 1953. Alzheimer's disease: a clinoco-pathologic analysis of twenty-three cases with a theory on pathogenesis. J Nerv Ment Dis. 118:97.

Hughes JT, Oppenheimer DR. 1969. Superficial siderosis of the central nervous system. A report on nine cases with autopsy. Acta Neuropathol (Berl). 13:56-74.

Miyasaki K, Murao S, Koizumi N. 1977. Hemochromatosis associated with brain lesions: a disorder of trace-metal binding proteins and/or polymers? J Neuropathol Exp Neurol. 36:664-76.

Rojas G, Messen L. 1968. Generalized cytosiderosis in two cases of progressive myoclonic epilepsy with Lafora inclusion bodies. Histopathological and ultrastructural studies. Neurocirugia. 26:3-11.

Vecchiola A, Asenjo A, Varleta J, Weinstein V, Oberhauser I. 1966.

[Iron in the blood, cerebrospinal fluid and urine in patients with Parkinson's disease and in patients without this disorder (primary report).] Neurocirugia. 24(3):129-30. Spanish.

1980-1989

Campbell KA, Bank B, Milgram NW. 1984. Epileptogenic effects of electrolytic lesions in the hippocampus: role of iron deposition. Exp Neurol. 86:506-14.

Cohen G. 1984. Oxy-radical toxicity in catecholamine neurons. Neurotoxicology. 5(1)77-82.

Craelius W, Migdal MW, Luessenhop CP, Sugar A, Mihalakis I. 1982. Iron deposits surrounding multiple sclerosis plaques. Arch Pathol Lab Med. 106:397-99.

Dexter DT, Wells FR, Lees AJ, Agid F, Agid Y, Jenner P, Marsden CD. 1989. Increased nigral iron content and alterations in other metal ions occurring in brain in Parkinson's disease. J Neurochem. 52:1830-6.

Jenner P. 1989. Clues to the mechanism underlying dopamine cell death in Parkinson's disease. J Neurol Neurosurg Psychiatry. Suppl:22-8.

Jones HJ, Hedley WE. 1983. Idiopathic hemochromatosis (IHC): dementia and ataxia as presenting signs. Neurology. 33:1479-83.

Koeppen AH, Barron KD, Csiza CK, Greenfield EA. 1988. Comparative immunocytochemistry of Palizaeus-Merzbacher disease, the jimpy mouse, and the myelin-deficient rat. J Neurol Sci. 84:315-27.

Langston JW. 1988. Neuromelanin-containing neurons are selectively vulnerable in parkinsonism. Trends Pharmacol Sci. 9(10):347-8.

Riederer P, Sofic E, Rausch WD, Schmidt B, Reynolds GP, Jellinger K, Youdim MB. 1989. Transition metals, ferritin, glutathione, and ascorbic acid in parkinsonian brains. J Neurochem. 52(2):515-20.

Sofic E, Riederer P, Heinsen H, Beckmann H, Reynolds GP, Hebenstreit G, Youdim MB. 1988. Increased iron (III) and total iron content in post mortem substantia nigra of parkinsonian brain. J Neural Transm. 74:199-205.

Thompson CM, Marksberry WR, Ehmann WD, Mao YY, Vance DE. 1988. Regional brain trace-element studies in Alzheimer's disease. Neurotoxicology. 9:1.

Valk J. 1989. *Magnetic Resonance of Myelin, Myelination and Myelin Disorders.* New York: Springer-Verlag.

Youdim MB, Ben-Shachar D, Riederer P. 1980. Is Parkinson's disease a progressive siderosis of substantia nigra resulting in iron and melanin induced neurodegeneration? Acta Neurol Scand Suppl. 126:47-54.

Youdim MB, Ben-Shachar D, Riederer P. 1989. Is Parkinson's disease a progressive siderosis of substantia nigra resulting in iron and melanin induced neurodegeneration? Acta Neurol Scand Suppl. 126:47-54.

1990-1999

Bartzokis G, Cummings J, Perlman S, Hance DB, Mintz J. 1999. Increased basal ganglia iron levels in Huntington disease. Arch Neurol. 56(5):569-74.

Ben-Shachar D, Eshel G, Finberg JP, Youdim MB. 1991. The iron chelator desferrioxamine (Desferal) retards 6-hydroxydopamine-induced degeneration of nigrostriatal dopamine neurons. J Neurochem. 56(4):1441-4.

Ben-Shachar D, Eshel G, Riederer P, Youdim MB. 1992. Role of iron and iron chelation in dopaminergic-induced neurodegeneration: implication for Parkinson's disease. Ann Neurol. 32 Suppl:S105-10.

Ben-Shachar D, Riederer P, Youdim MB. 1991. Iron-melanin interaction and lipid peroxidation: implications for Parkinson's disease. J Neurochem. 57(5):1609-14.

Ben-Shachar D, Youdim MB. 1990. Selectivity of melaninized nigrastriatal dopamine neurons to degeneration in Parkinson's disease may depend on iron-melanin interaction. J Neural Transm Suppl. 29:251-8.

———— 1991. Intranigral iron injection induces behavioral and biochemical "parkinsonism" in rats. J Neurochem. 57(6):2133-5.

———— 1993. Iron, melanin and dopamine interaction: relevance to Parkinson's disease. Prog Neuropsychopharmacol Biol Psychiatry. 17(1):139-50.

Bentur Y, Koren G, Tesoro A, Carley H, Olivien N, Freedman MH. 1990. Comparison of deferoxamine pharmacokinetics between asymptomatic thalassemic children and those exhibiting severe neurotoxicity. Clin Pharmacol Ther. 47(4):478-82.

Berg D, Grote C, Rausch WD, Maurer M, Wesemann W, Riederer P, Becker G. 1999. Iron accumulation in the substantia nigra in rats visualized by ultrasound. Ultrasound Med Biol. 25(6):901-4.

Blass JP, Gibson GE. 1991. The role of oxidative abnormalities in the pathophysiology of Alzheimer's disease. Rev Neurol. 147:513.

Carlsson A, Fornstedt B. 1991. Possible mechanism underlying the special vulnerability of dopaminergic neurons. Acta Neurol Scand Suppl. 136:16-18.

Connor JR, Menzies SL, St. Martin S, Fine RE, Mufson EJ. 1991. Altered cellular distribution of transferrin, ferritin and iron in Alzheimer's disease brains. J Neurosci Res. 31:75.

Connor JR, Menzies ST, St Martin SM, Mufson EJ. 1992a. A histochemical study of iron, transferrin, and ferritin in Alzheimer's diseased brains. J Neurosci Res. 1992. 31(1):75-83.

Connor JR, Snyder BS, Beard JL, Fine RE, Mufson EJ. 1992b. The regional distribution of iron and iron regulatory proteins in the brain in aging and Alzheimer's disease. J Neurosci Res. 31:327.

Connor JR. 1992. Proteins of iron regulation in the brain in Alzheimer's disease. In Lauffer RB, ed. 1992. *Iron and Human Disease.* Ann Arbor, MI: CRC Press, pp 54-67.

Cutler P. 1994. Iron overload an psychiatric illness. Can J Psychiatry. 39:8-11.

Dexter DT, Carayon A, Javoy-Agid F, Agid Y, Wells FR, Daniel SE, Lees AJ, Jenner P, Marsden CD. 1991 Alterations if nte levels of iron, ferritin and other trace metals in Parkinson's disease and other neurodegenerative diseases affecting the basal ganglia. Brain. 114:1953-75.

Double KL, Riederer PF, Gerlach M. 1999. Role of iron in 6-hydroxydopamine neurotoxicity. Adv Neurol. 80:287-96.

Ebadu NM, Srinivasan SK, Baxi MD. 1996. Oxidative stress and antioxidant therapy in Parkinson's disease. Prog Neurobiol. 48(1):1-19.

Enochs WS, Sarna T, Zecca L, Swatz HM. 1994. The roles of neuromelanin, binding of metal ions, and oxidative cytotoxicity in the pathogenesis of Parkinson's disease: a hypothesis. J Neural Transm Park Dis Dement Sect. 7(2): 83-100.

Fahn S, Cohen G. 1992. The oxidant stress hypothesis in Parkinson's disease: evidence supporting it. Ann Neurol. 32(6):804-12.

Faucheux BA, Hirsch BC. 1998. [Iron homeostasis and Parkinson's disease.] Ann Biol Clin (Paris). 56 Spec No: 23-30.

Galazka-Friedman J, Friedman A. 1997. Controversies about iron in parkinsonian and control substantia nigra. Acta Neurobiol Exp (Wars). 57(3):217-225.

Gelman BB, Rodriguz-Wolf MS, Wen J. 1992. Siderotic cerebral macrophages in aquired immunodeficiency syndrome. Arch Pathol Lab Med. 116:509.

Gocht A, Lohler J. 1990. Changes in glial cell markers in recent and old demyelating lesions in central pontine myelinolysis. Acta Neuropathol. 80:46-58.

Good PF, Olanow CW, Perl DP. 1992. Neuromelanin-containing neurons of the substantia nigra accumulate iron and aluminum in Parkinson's disease; a LAMMA study. Brain res. 593(2):343-6.

Gotz ME, Freyberger A, Riederer P. 1990. Oxidative stress: a role in the pathogenesis of Parkinson's disease. J eural Transm Suppl. 29:241-9.

Griffiths PD, Crossman AR. 1993. Distribution of iron in the basal ganglia and neocortex in postmortem tissue in Parkinson's disease and Alzheimer's disease. Dementia. 4(2):61-5.

Hall S, Rutledge JN, Schallert T. 1992. MRI, brain iron and experimental Parkinson's disease. J Neurol Sci. 113(2):198-208.

Han J, Cheng FC, Yang Z, Dryhurst G. 1999. Inhibitors of mitochondrial respiration, Iron (II), and hydroxyl radical evoke release and extracellular hydrolysis of glutathione in the rat striatum and substantia nigra: potential implications to Parkinson's disease. J Neurochem. 73(4): 1683-95.

Hirsch EC. 1993. Does oxidative stress participate in nerve cell death in Parkinson's disease? Eur Neurol. 33 Suppl 1:52-9.

———— 1994. Biochemistry of Parkinson's disease with special reference to the dopaminergic systems. Mol Neurobiol. 9(1-3): 135-42.

Jellinger K, Kienzl E, Rumpelmair G, Riederer P, Stachelberger H, Ben-Shachar D, Youdin MB. 1992. Iron-melanin complex in substantia nigra of parkinsonian brains: an x-ray microanalysis. J Neurochem. 59(3):1168-71.

Jellinger K, Paulus W, Guundke-Iqbal I, Riederer P, Youdim MB. 1990. Brain iron ferritin in Parkinson's and Alzheimer's disease. J Neural Transm Park Dis Dement Sect.2(4):327-40.

Jellinger KA. 1999. The role of iron in neurodegeneration: prospects for pharmacotherapy of Parkinson's disease. Drugs Aging. 14(2):115-40.

Jenner P, Olanow CW. 1996. Oxidative stress and the pathogenesis of Parkinson's disease. Neurology. 47(6 Suppl 3):S161-70.

Jenner P, Schapira AH, Marsden CD. 1992. New insights into the cause of Parkinson's disease. Neurology. 42(12):2241-50.

Jenner P. 1991. Oxidative stress as a cause of Parkinson's disease. Acta Neurol Scand Suppl. 136:6-15.

Jenner P. 1992. What process causes nigral cell death in Parkinson's disease? Neurol Clin. 10(2):387-403.

———— 1993. Altered mitochondrial function, iron metabolism and glutathione levels in Parkinson's disease. Acta Neurol Scand Suppl. 146:6-13.

———— 1993. Presymptomatic detection of Parkinson's disease. J Neural Transm Suppl. 40:23-36.

———— 1998. Oxidative mechanisms in nigral cell death in Parkinson's disease. Mov Disord. 13 Suppl 1: 24-34.

Kienzl E, Jellinger K, Stachelberger H, Linert W. 1999. Iron as a catalyst for oxidative stress in the pathogenesis of Parkinson's disease? Life Sci. 65(18-19):1973-6.

Kienzl E, Puchinger L, Jellinger K, Linert W, Stachelberger H, Jameson RF. 1995. The role of transition metals in the pathogenesis of Parkinson's disease. J Neurol Sci. 134 Suppl: 69-78.

Loeffler DA, Connor JR, Juneau PL, Snyder BS, Kanaley L, De Maggio AJ, Nguyen H, Brickman CM, LeWitt PA. 1995. Transferrin and iron in normal, Alzheimer's disease, and Parkinson's disease regions. J Neurochem. 66(2):710-24.

Mann VM, Cooper JM, Daniel SE, Srai K, Jenner P, Marsden CD, Schapira AH. 1995. Complex I, iron, and ferritin in Parkinson's disease substantia nigra. Ann Neurol. 36(6): 875-8.

Montgomery EG Jr. 1995. Heavy metals and the etiology of Parkinson's disease and other movement disorders. Toxicology. 97(1-3):3-9.

Morris CM, Edwardson JA. 1994. Iron histochemistry of the substantia nigra in Parkinson's disease. Neurodegeneration. 3(4):277-82.

Nakano M. 1993. A possible mechanism of iron neurotoxicity. Eur Neurol. 33 Suppl:44-51.

Nielsen JE, Jensen LN, Drabbe K. 1995. Hereditary haemochromatosis: a case of iron accumulating in the basal ganglia associated with a parkinsonian syndrome. J Neurol Neurosurg Psychiatry. 59:318-21.

Olanow CW, Marsden D, Perl D, Cohen G, eds. 1992. *Iron and Oxidative Stress in Parkinson's Disease*. Ann Neurol. 32:Suppl.

Olanow CW. 1992. An introduction to the free radical hypothesis in Parkinson's disease. Ann Neurol. 32 Suppl:S2-9.

Owen AD, Schapira AH, Jenner P, Marsden CD. 1996. Oxidative stress and Parkinson's disease. Ann N Y Acad Sci. 12(1):73-94.

Riederer P, Lange KW. 1992. Pathogenesis of Parkinson's disease. Curr Opin Neurol Neurosurg. 5(3):1080-9.

Sengstock GJ, Olanow CW, Dunn AJ, Arendash GW. 1992. Iron induces degeneration of nigrostriatal neurons. Brain Res Bull. 28(4):645-9.

Smith Sl, Maggs JL, Edwards G, Ward SA, Park BK, McLean WG. 1998. The role of iron in neurotoxicity: a study of novel antimalarial drugs.

Neurotoxicity. 19(4-5):557-9.

Sofic E, Paulus W, Jellinger K, Riederer P, Youdim MB. 1991. Selective increase of iron in substantia nigra zona compacta of parkinsonian brains. J Neurochem. 56(3):978-82.

Swaiman KF. 1991. Hallervorden-Spatz syndrome and brain iron metabolism. Arch Neurol. 48:1285-93.

Tanaka M, Sotomatsu A, Kanai H, Hirai S. 1991. Dopa and dopamine caused cultured neuronal death in the presence of iron. J Neurol Sci. 101(2):198-203.

Temlett JA, Landsberg JP, Watt F, Grime GW. 1994. Increased iron in the substantis nigra compacta of the MPTP-lesioned hemiparkinsonian African green monkey: evidence from proton microprobe elemental microanalysis. J Neurochem. 62(1):134-46.

Yantin F, Andersen JK. 1999. The role of iron in Parkinson disease and 1-methyl-4-phenyl-1,2,3,6-tehydropyridine toxicity. IUBMB Life. 48(2):139-41.

Yodim MB, Ben-Schachar D, Riederer P. 1993. The possible role of iron in the etiopathology of Parkinson's disease. Mov Disord. 8(1):1-12.

———— 1991. Iron in brain function and dysfunction with emphasis on Parkinson's disease. Eur Neurol. 31 Suppl 1:34-40.

———— 1990. The role of monoamine oxidase, iron-melanin interaction, and intracellular calcium in Parkinson's disease. J Neural Transm Suppl. 32:239-48.

Youdim MB, Ben-Shachar D, Eshel G, Finberg JP, Riederer P. 1993. The neurotoxicity of iron and nitric oxide. Relevance to the etiology of Parkinson's disease. Adv Neurol. 60:259-66.

Youdim MB, Riederer P. 1993. The role of iron in senescence of dopamiergic neurons in Parkinson's disease. J Neural Transm Suppl. 40:57-67.

2000-2007

Amit T, Avramovich-Tirosh Y, Youdim MB, Mandel S. 2007. Targeting multiple Alzheimer's disease etiologies with multimodal neuroprotective and neurorestorative iron chelators. FASEB. [Epub ahead of print] PMID: 18048580.

Anderson JK. 2001. Do alterations in glutathione and iron levels contribute to pathology associated with Parkinson's disease? Novartis Found Symp. 235:11-20.

———— 2004. Iron dysregulation and Parkinson's disease. J Alzheimer's Dis. 6(6 Suppl):547-52.

Bartzokis G, Tishler TA, Shin IS, Lu PH, Cummingl JL. 2004 Brain ferritin iron as a risk factor for age at onset in neurodegerative diseases. Ann N Y Acad Sci. 1012:221-36.

Bartzokis G, Tishler TA. 2000. MRI evaluation of basal ganglia ferritin iron and neurotoxicity in Alzheimer's and Huntington's disease. Cell Mol Biol (Noisy-le-grand). 46(4):821-33.

Berg D, Hochstrasser H, Schweitzer KJ, Riess O. 2006. Disturbance of iron metabolism in Parkinson's disease – ultrasonography as a biomarker. Neurotox Res. 9(1):1-13.

Bharath S, Hsu M, Kaur D, Rajagopalan S, Anderson JK. 2002. Glutathione, iron and Parkinson's disease. Biochem Pharmacol 64(5-6): 1037-48.

Borg D. 2006. In vivo detection of iron and neuromelanin by transcranial sonography – a new approach for early detection of substantia nigra damage. PMID: 16755382.

Brewer GJ. 2007. Iron and copper toxicity in diseases of aging, particularly atherosclerosis and Alzheimer's disease. Exp Biol Med (Maywowd). 232(2):323-35.

Castellani RJ, Honda K, Zhu X, Cash AD, Nunomura A, Perry G, Smith MA. 2004. Contribution of redox-active iron and copper to oxidative damage in Alzheimer disease. Ageing Res Rev. 3:319-26.

Castellani RJ, Siedlak SL, Perry G, Smith MA. 2000. Sequestration of iron by Lewy bodies in Parkinson's disease. Acta Neuroathol (Berl). 100(2):111-4.

Cheung PT. 2007. Iron, sense and neurotoxicity. Hong Kong Med J. 13(5):412.

Chwiej J, Adamek D, Szczerbowska-Boruchowska M, Krygowska-Wajs A, Wojcik S Falenberg G, Manka A, Lankosz M. 2007. Investigations of differences in iron oxidation state inside single neurons from substantia nigra of Parkinson's disease and control patients using the micro-XANES technique. J Biol Inorg Chem. 12(2)204-11.

Collins MA, Neafsey EJ. 2002. Potential neurotoxic "agents provocateurs" in Parkinson's disease. Neurotoxidol Teratol. 24(5):571-7.

Dobson J. 2004. Magnetic iron compounds in neurological disorders. Ann NY Acad Sci. 1012:183-92.

Double KL, Ben-Shacar D, Youdim MB, Zecca I, Riederer P, Gerlach M. 2002. Influence of neuromelanin on oxidative pathways within the human substantia nigra. Neurotoxicol Teratol. 24(5):621-8.

Double KL, Gerlach M, Schuneman V, Trautwein AX, Zecca L, Gallorini M, Youdim MB, Riederer P, Ben-Schacher D. 2003. Iron-binding characteristics of neuromelanin of the human substantia nigra. Biochem Pharmacol. 66(3): 489-94.

Double KL, Gerlach M, Youdim MB, Riederer P. 2000. Impaired iron homeostasis in Parkinson's disease. J Neural Transm Suppl. 37-58.

Faucheux BA, Martin ME, Beaumont C, Hauw JJ, Agrid Y, Hirsch BC. 2003. Neuromelanin associated redox-active iron is increased in the substantia nigra of patients with Parkinson's disease. J Neurochem. 86(5): 1142-8.

Floor E. 2000. Iron as a vulnerability factor in nigrostriatal degeneration in aging and Parkinson's disease. Cell Mol Biol (Noisy-le-grand). 46(4): 709-20.

Gal S, Fridkin M, Amit T, Aheng H, Youdim MB. 2006. M30, a novel multifunctional neuroprotective drug with potent iron chelating and brain selective monoamine oxidase-ab inhibitory activity for Parkinsonson's disease. Neural Transm Suppl. 70:447-56.

Gerlach M, Bouble KL, Ben-Shachar D, Zecca L, Youdim MB, Riederer P. 2003. Neuromelanin and its interaction with iron as a potential risk factor for dopaminergic neurodegeneration underlying Parkinson's disease. Neurotox Res. 5(1-2):35-44.

Grunblatt E, Mandel S, Youdim MB. 2000. Neuroprotective strategies in Parkinson's disease using the models of 6-hydroxydopamine and MPTP. Ann N Y Acad Sci. 899:262-73.

Hirsch EC. 2006. Altered regulation of iron transport and storage in Parkinson's disease. J Neural Transm Suppl. 71: 201-4.

Honda K, Casadesus G, Petersen RB, Perry G, Smith MA. 2004. Oxidative stress and redox-active iron in Alzheimer's disease. Ann N Y Acad Sci 1012:179-82.

Ikeda M. 2001. Iron overload without the C282Y mutation in patients with epilepsy. J Neurol Neurosurg Psychiatry. 70:551-53.

Izumi Y, Sawada H, Sakka N, Yamamoto N, Kume T, Katsuki H, Shimohama S, Akaike A. 2005. p-Quinone mediates 6-hydroxydopamine-induced dopaminergic neuronal death and ferrous iron accelerates the conversion of p-quinone into melanin extracellularly. J Neurosci Res 79(6):849-60.

Jiang H, Song N, Wang J, Ren Ly, Xie JX. 2007. Peripheral iron dextran induced degeneration of dopaminergic neurons in rat substantia nigra. Neurochem Int. 51(1):32-6.

Kaur D, Anderson JK. 2002. Ironing out Parkinson's disease: is therapeutic treatment with iron chelators a real possibility? Aging Cell. 1(1):17-21.

Lange, AE. 2007. The progression of Parkinson disease: a hypothesis. Neurology. 68(2):948-52.

Levine SM, Chakrabarty A. 2004. The role of iron in the pathogenesis of experimental allergic encephalomyelitis and multiple sclerosis. Ann NY Acad Sci. 1012:252-66.

Maharaj DS, Maharaj H, Daya S, Glass BD. 2006. Melatonin and 6-hydroxymelatonin protect against iron-induced neurotoxicity. J Neurochem 96(1):78-81.

Michaeli S, Oz G, Source DJ, Garwood M, Ugurbil K, Majestic S, Tuite P. 2007. Assessment of brain iron and neuronal integrity in patients with Parkinson's disease using novel MRI contrasts. Mov Disord. 22(3):334-40..

Oakley AE, Collingwood JF, Dobson J, Love G, Perrott HR, Edwardson JA, Elstner M, Morris CM. 2007. Individual dopaminergic neurons show raised iron levels in Parkinson disease. Neurology. 68:1820-25.

Ortega R, Cloetens P, Deves G, Carmona A, Bohics. 2007. Iron storage within dopamine neurovesicles revealed by chemical nano-imaging. PLoS ONE. 2(9)e925.

Rouault TA, Cooperman S. 2006. Brain iron metabolism. Semin Pediatr Neurol. 13(3):142-8.

Salazar J, Mena N, Nunez MT. 2006. Iron dyshomeostasis in Parkinson's disease. J Neural Transm Suppl. 71:205-13.

Selim MH, Ratan RR. 2004. The role of iron neurotoxicity in ischemic stroke. 2004. Ageing Res Rev. 3(3):345-53.

Shoham S, Youdim MB. 2004. Nutritional iron deprivation attenuates kainite-induced neurotoxicity in rats: implications for involvement of iron in neurodegeneration. Ann N Y Acad Sci. 1012:94-114.

Stankiewicz J, Panter SS, Neema M, Arora A, Batt CE, Bakshi R. 2007. Iron in chronic brain disorders: imaging and neurotherapeutic implications. Neurotherapeutics. 4(3):37-86.

Sulzer D, Schmitz Y. 2007. Parkinson's disease: return of an old prime suspect. Neuron. 55:8-10.

Takanashi M, Mochizuki H, Yokomizo K, Hattori N, Mori H, Yamamura Y, Mizuno Y. 2001. Iron accumulation in the substantia nigra of autosomal recessive juvenile parkinsonism (ARJJP). Parkinsonism Relat Disord. 7(4):311-13.

Todorich BM, Connor JR. 2004. Redox metals in Alzheimer's disease. Ann NY Acad Sci. 1012:171-78.

Wersinger C, Sidhu A. 2006. An inflammatory pathomechanism for Parkinson's disease? Curr Med Chem. 13(5):591-602.

Whitton, PS. 2007. Inflammation as a causative factor in the aetiology of Parkinson's disease. Br J Pharmacol. 150(8):963-76.

Wright RO, Baccarelli A. 2007. Metals and neurotoxicology. J Nutr. 137(12):2809-13.

Yoo MS, Chun HS, Son JJ, DiGiorgio LA, Kim DJ, Peng C, Son JH. 2003. Oxidative stress regulated genes in nigral dopaminergic neuronal cells: correlation with the known pathology in Parkinson's disease. Brain Res Mol Brain Res   110(1): 76-84.

Youdim MB, Fridkin M, Zheng H. 2004. Novel bifunctional drugs targeting monoamine oxidase inhibition and iron chelation as an approach to neuroprotection in Parkinson's disease and other neurodegenerative diseases. J Neural Transm. 111:1455-71.

———— 2005. Bifunctional drug derivatives of MAO-B inhibitor rasagiline and iron chelator VK-28 as a more effective approach to treatment of brain ageing in ageing neurodegenerative diseases. Mech Ageing Dev. 126:317-26.

Youdim MB, Stephenson G, Ben-Shachar D. 2004. Ironing iron out in Parkinson's disease and other neurodegenerative diseases with iron chelators: a lesson from 6-hydroxydopamine and iron chelators, desferal and VK-28. Ann N Y Acad Sci. 1012:306-25.

Youdim MB. 2003. What we have learnt from CDNA microarray gene expression studies about the role of iron in MPTP induced neurodegeneration and Parkinson's disease? J Neural Transm Suppl. (65):73-88.

Xudong H, Moir RD, Tanzi RE, Bush AL, Rogers JT. 2004. Redox-active metals, oxidative stress, and Alzheimer's disease pathology. Ann NY Acad Sci. 1012:153-63.

Zecca L, Youdim MBH, Riederer P, Conner JR, Crichton, RR. 2004. Iron, brain ageing and neurodegenerative disorders. Nature Reviews Neuroscience. 5:863-73.

Zucca FA, Bellei C, Gianelli S, Terreni MR, Gallorini M, Rizzio G, Albertini A, Zecca L. 2006. Neuromelanin and iron in human locus coeruleus and substantia nigra during aging: consequences for neuronal vulnerability. J Neural Transm. 113(6):757-67.

Chapter 6

Carcinogenicity of Iron Compounds

Introduction

Cancer development takes place in three phases: 1) Initiation; 2) Promotion; and 3) Progression. With the exception of iron, all carcinogens act either in initiation or promotion. However, iron is a unique carcinogen because iron acts on all three phases. By way of redox cycling, which generates the hydroxyl radical, iron participates in the initiation and promotional phases of cancer development.

Once the promoted cancer cells aggregate to form a tumor, they develop a voracious appetite for iron, demonstrated by the development of large numbers of transferrin receptors. Recall that transferrin is the transport protein for iron—transferrin delivers iron to cells that display transferrin receptors on their surface; the more transferrin receptors a cell has, the more iron the cell can scavenge. Because cancer cells have many more receptors on their surface, they deprive adjacent cells of iron, causing an area of iron-deficient, anemic cells surrounding the tumor. In this way, the tumor is able to invade and conquer. Pretty good strategy—starve the enemy and then destroy it!

The gist of this is that iron is the only known substance that participates in all three phases of cancer development: initiation, promotion, and progression. For this reason, it is necessary to develop new nomenclature to describe iron's carcinogenicity. Because iron is involved in all three phases of carcinogenesis, iron should be identified as the only known "Complete Carcinogen."

However, iron's carcinogenic effects go even beyond those that are implied by the term, "Complete Carcinogen." Perhaps iron is better identified as "The Ultimate Carcinogen," because, in addition to acting in the three phases of cancer development:

- Iron activates xenobiotics ("foreign chemicals"), turning them into carcinogens.
- Iron is a factor leading to alcoholic liver cirrhosis, a precursor to liver cancer in alcoholics.
- Iron acts synergistically with viral infections (hepatitis C, hepatitis B, HIV, Papillomavirus) in causing cancer.
- Iron multiplies aflatoxin carcinogenicity. Aflatoxin is a liver carcinogen that is produced by a fungus, therefore called a mycotoxin. Other mycotoxins are also synergistically carcinogenic with iron.
- Iron plays a critical role in causing cancer cells to become more aggressive and invasive, and to spread to other sites (metastasize).

We could also refer to iron and oxygen as the Original Mutagens (OMs), because, through their mutual interaction, iron and oxygen have directed evolution from the first primitive iron/oxygen-utilizing organisms to the vast array of animal, plant, and microbial life that exists today. Iron and oxygen are the yin and yang of evolution.

Carcinogenicity of Iron in the 2001 DRIs

At the time the 2001 DRIs (Food and Nutrition Board 2001) were being formulated, the published medical and scientific literature that identified iron as a human carcinogen was extensive. Currently, it is so vast that no individual can even come close to reviewing all of it. Nevertheless, the section on *Cancer* in the *Hazard Identification* in the 2001 DRIs (pp 370-372) consisted of five short paragraphs and cited only 10 references! Big Brother decided to continue forcing iron-adulterated food on the North American population without even considering a small fraction of the published literature regarding the carcinogenicity of iron compounds.

Iron is a Carcinogen

It may seem strange to many that it is possible to categorically state that iron is a carcinogen. Because iron is crucial to our lives, most people are surprised to hear this. What is the basis for such a bold statement? Are the carcinogenic properties of iron fact or fiction? In this chapter, we will examine the evidence that should convince even the greatest skeptic that iron's potential for causing cancer, when injected, inhaled, or consumed, is very real, and should not be blown off in five short paragraphs by the people who have promised to guard the nutritional health of residents of the United States.

Follow the Evidence

The evidence linking iron to cancer proceeds along several lines, including toxicology, clinical observation, and epidemiology. "Follow the Evidence," the theme of the famous CSI television series, is also the theme of this chapter, and, in fact this entire book. We will examine the evidence, and it will be demonstrated beyond reasonable doubt that iron is capable of damaging DNA and causes cancer in animals and humans. In view of the vast documentation, only a fraction of which is presented here, the Food and Nutrition Board must be severely chastised. The failure to provide a sound evaluation of the carcinogenic potential of iron is irresponsible, and places the entire North American population at risk for the damaging effects resulting from the continuing adulteration of our food supply by the addition of a wide variety of iron-containing compounds.

Mutagen testing has demonstrated mutagenicity for a variety of iron compounds that are added to food (Dunkel et al. 1999). Table 5 lists the iron compounds certified by the FDA for use in foods. Animal testing has demonstrated carcinogenicity of all of these iron compounds. As well, when excess iron accumulates in the liver, as happens in hereditary hemochromatosis, African siderosis, and other iron overload conditions, liver cancer is frequently a fatal consequence. Hepatitis C, hepatitis B, and HIV viral infections are increased among people with high iron levels, and may also result in various forms of cancer.

Table 5. Iron Compounds Certified for Use in Food[a]

Ferric [Fe(III)]	Ferrous [Fe(II)]	Reduced Iron [Fe(o)]	Other Forms of Iron
1. ammonium citrate	8. ascorbate	15. elemental iron	18. iron-choline citrate
2. chloride	9. carbonate	16. electrolytic iron	19. iron-deferroxamine
3. citrate	10. citrate	17. iron carbonyl	20. iron oxide[c]
4. phosphate	11. fumarate		
5. pyrophosphate	12. gluconate		
6. sulfate	13. lactate		
7. sodium pyrophosphate	14. sulfate[b]		

[a]Adapted from Food and Nutrition Board (1993), p 119.
[b]Also approved for use as a "flavoring agent."
[c]Used as coloring agent (red/orange).

There is conflicting epidemiology regarding the role of heme iron and/or elevated body levels of stored iron in cancer. However, when viewed in light of the proven mutagenicity and carcinogenicity of iron-containing compounds, the epidemiology that indicates increased cancer incidence associated with increased iron consumption and increased body iron burden should be accepted as a very real possibility.

Testing the Hypothesis

In toxicology, two major criteria are used for establishing the carcinogenicity of any substance. These involve: 1) Testing various human or animal cell lines to determine if the substance can cause DNA strand breakage or other evidence of DNA damage; 2) Testing laboratory animals to determine if the substance can cause cancer in laboratory animals.

If the toxicology indicates that a substance is mutagenic and animal models demonstrate that the substance causes cancer, clinical evidence of the relationship between that substance and cancer in humans must be examined. If there is both toxicological and clinical evidence that a substance is carcinogenic, the statistical methods of epidemiology are used to try to sort out the details. An approximate outline for testing the hypothesis that iron is carcinogenic might be as follows.

- Toxicology
  o Does iron induce mutations in established human or animal cell lines?
  o Does iron cause cancer in laboratory animals?
- Clinical Observations / Epidemiology
  o Do elevated iron levels result in an increase in cancer incidence?
    - Do people with hereditary iron overload have an increased incidence of cancer?
    - Do people with high dietary intake of iron have an increased incidence of cancer?
    - Does elevated serum ferritin indicate increased cancer risk?
    - Is elevated transferrin loading a predictor of cancer risk?
  o What is the relationship between iron, viral infection, and cancer?
    - Do increased iron stores predispose to hepatitis B-related liver cancer?
    - Are increased iron stores associated with hepatitis C-related liver cancer?
    - Are increased iron stores related to cancer incidence in people infected with human immunodeficiency virus (HIV)?
  o Genetic Evidence:
    - What is the role of hemochromatosis gene mutations

in cancer incidence?
- Are there other hereditary iron loading conditions that result in an increased incidence of cancer?
  o Dietary Evidence:
    - Can high dietary iron alone cause cancer in laboratory animals?
    - Is a diet high in red meat and/or other sources of iron associated with an increased incidence of cancer?
    - Does high dietary iron increase the carcinogenicity of other carcinogens?

As we follow the evidence, it will become abundantly clear that most cancers are, indeed, associated with increased body iron burden as indicated by increased transferrin loading and serum ferritin, as well as increased liver iron burden revealed by liver biopsy.

Inhalation Toxicology

"The association between inhalation of industrial sources of iron and development of respiratory tract neoplasias is well established."   (Weinberg 1996a)

The first indication of iron's carcinogenicity is that of Dreyfus (1936), who reported lung cancer in two siblings subsequent to inhaling iron oxide. The female sibling developed lung cancer at age 44, and the male at age 36. Dreyfus was interested in the cause of lung cancer in these two individuals because it was rare for lung cancer to develop at such an early age, and especially in two siblings. On investigation, Dreyfus learned that the siblings' mother worked at home when they were young children, polishing screws with iron oxide.

Additional evidence for carcinogenicity of iron compounds was accumulating in the same time period. Metal finishing workers in the British steel industry in Sheffield in 1926-35 had an increased incidence of cancers of the larynx, bronchial tubes, and lungs (Turner and Grace 1938). Turner and Grace reported that mortality from respiratory tract cancers were increased 2.4-fold among steel foundry and furnace workers, 2.0-fold among metal grinders, glazers and buffers, and 1.8-fold among steel machinists and turners, as compared to males in other occupations. Underground hematite miners in Cumberland (UK) were twice as likely to die of lung cancer as were persons who worked at the surface of the mines or who were coal miners (Boyd et al. 1970). A 5-16 fold increase in lung cancer mortality among underground iron ore miners, as compared with non-miners, was observed in Sweden (Edling 1982), and a 5-12 fold increase in Loraine (Antoine et al. 1979). In eastern Slovakia, the relative risk of lung cancer in iron ore minors, as compared with non-minors, was 2.81 in one district and 4.01 in a second district (Icso et al. 1994).

Campbell (1940) observed that mice exposed to ferric oxide dust during their early months of life develop malignant lung tumors as they age. Control mice exposed to silica dust without ferric oxide develop only a small number of nonmalignant tumors (refer to Weinberg 1996a for an excellent review of inhalation toxicology of iron compounds).

These early findings lay dormant for two decades when the next indication of iron's carcinogenicity surfaced with the introduction of iron dextran. We will return to the carcinogenicity of inhaled iron, and to the increased incidence of cancer in people with iron overload conditions after discussing iron dextran—the first iron compound officially classified as "reasonably anticipated to be a human carcinogen" (IARC 1973).

Iron Dextran

"One might worry about the iron-injectable compounds which are being tested and used. One could almost guess that someone is going to find iron dextran carcinogenic."
(Furst 1960)

Iron dextran is a complex of ferric hydroxide with dextran, a polysaccharide. The iron dextran complex is very soluble in water and insoluble in most organic solvents. The property of water solubility makes iron dextran ideal for use by injection. Iron dextran complex was introduced in the United States in 1957 (IARC 1973).

In 1959, Richmond (1959) reported the induction of sarcoma in rats by iron dextran. In 1960, Robinson et al. (1960) reported a human case of malignant neoplasm developing at the site of injection of iron dextran. A number of studies rapidly confirmed the carcinogenicity of iron dextran in laboratory animals and humans (Richmond 1960a, 1960b; Schulman 1960; Haddow and Horning 1960; Crowley and Still 1960; Muir and Goldberg 1961; Viallier and Rebouillat 1962; Roe and Lancaster 1964; Haddow et al. 1964; Gillie 1964; Thedering 1964; Roe et al. 1964; Giuffrida et al. 1964; Kunz 1964; Chandra 1965; Roe and Carter 1967; Carter et al. 1968; Carter 1969).

In 1973, IARC stated, "Iron dextran complex is *reasonably anticipated to be a human carcinogen* based on sufficient evidence of carcinogenicity in experimental animals." Iron dextran complex was first listed as "reasonably anticipated to be a human carcinogen" in the Second Annual Report on Carcinogens (Report on Carcinogens 1981). The carbohydrate, dextran, alone is not carcinogenic. We have followed the evidence and can conclude beyond reasonable doubt: Iron dextran is a human carcinogen.

According to the Report on Carcinogens (2002) in the United States, "Iron dextran complex is used for parenteral treatment of iron-deficiency anemia, but is used only in special cases such as when oral treatment has failed. It is also used in veterinary medicine to treat baby pigs."

Iron Gluconate

"Playing with iron is almost literally playing with fire."
(Stevens 1992, p 344)

Iron gluconate is another water-soluble iron compound for potential use by injection and has largely replaced iron dextran in clinical settings in the U.S. The suggestion has been made that iron gluconate would be ideal for adding to milk. There is a lack of information in regard to iron gluconate. However, Carter et al. (1968)

demonstrated induction of tumors in mice and rats with both ferric sodium gluconate and iron dextran. Because iron gluconate may be used instead of iron dextran, Eichbaum et al. (2003) have addressed the question, "Is iron gluconate really safer that iron dextran?" There is no answer to this question at the present time. It is, however, very likely that iron gluconate as well as any other injectable form of iron will be carcinogenic. Additional studies are seriously needed.

Iron Dextran in Developing Countries

When will we ever learn? In India and other developing countries, iron dextran is being used on underprivileged women to treat moderate pregnancy anemia in routine prenatal care. Sharma et al. (2004) reported results of a partially randomized efficacy field trial comparing 100 daily oral doses of iron with 3 intramuscular iron dextran injections given at 1-month intervals for alleviation of pregnancy anemia in a public hospital setting in New Delhi. In an Editorial in the same issue of the American Journal of Clinical Nutrition, Solomons and Schümann (2004) question the ethics of this practice in an article entitled, "Intramuscular administration of iron dextran is inappropriate for treatment of moderate pregnancy anemia, both in intervention research on underprivileged women and in routine prenatal care provided by public health services." Nevertheless, the practice continues unabated.

Inhaled Iron

"Elimination of industrial use of crocidolite and amosite and of any chrysolite that is contaminated with iron or with iron-containing tremolite could lead to a striking reduction in asbestos-related cancer morbidity." (Weinberg 1989)

Asbestos refers to a group of hydrated fibrous silicates that have been widely used for insulation and industrial purposes. Asbestos mining and manufacture was begun in the 1890s. Large deposits of white asbestos (chrysolite) were found in Canada and Russia, while blue asbestos (crocidolite) was mined in South Africa. Early in the 1900s, a brown asbestos named amosite was found in South Africa. Later in the 1900s, after World War II, crocidolite was found in Western Australia and, to a limited extent, elsewhere. A white asbestos known as tremolite has been used in rural areas of Greece, Turkey, and Melanesia to paint houses.

The carcinogenic properties of asbestos are well known. We have all either lived in homes from which asbestos has been removed, or observed workers removing asbestos from public buildings. The suggestion that mesothelioma resulted from occupational exposure to asbestos was first made by Gloyne in Britain (Gloyne 1935). A comprehensive review, "The epidemiology of mesothelioma in historical context," is available (McDonald and McDonald 1996).

A case-control study in New Caledonia, where tremolite paint (locally named "pö") is used, examined cases diagnosed between 1993-1995, which included 15 pleural mesotheliomas, 228 lung cancers, and 23 laryngeal cancers, compared to 305 controls (Luce et al. 2000). All Melanesian cases had been exposed to whitewash. The risk of mesothelioma was strongly associated with whitewash. Among Melanesian women, exposure to whitewash was associated with lung cancer. Smokers exposed to whitewash had an approximately nine-fold increased risk compared with women who never smoked and had never used whitewash.

Crocidolite contains up to 27% iron by weight and is more carcinogenic in humans than chrysolite, which contains 2-3% iron by weight. Thus, it has been proposed that the iron from asbestos catalyzes the generation of reactive oxygen species that may play a role in the carcinogenicity of asbestos (Weinberg 1989).

Asbestos Carcinogenicity

The generation of reactive oxygen species as an explanation for the carcinogenicity of asbestos started accumulating in the mid-1980s, and continues right up to the present time (Wright et al. 1983; Warheit et al. 1984; Weitzman and Graceffa 1984; Donaldson and Cullen 1984; Donaldson et al. 1985; Elstner et al. 1986; Mossman et al. 1986; Koerten et al. 1986; Case et al. 1986; Goodglick and Kane

1986; Hansen and Mossman 1987; Turver and Brown 1987; Shatos et al. 1987; Elstner et al. 1988; Mossman and Marsh 1989; Iguchi and Kojo 1989; Churg. et al. 1989; Goodglick and Kane 1990; Koerten et al. 1990; Kamp et al. 1992, 1995; Nicholson and Raffn 1995; Xu et al. 1999, 2002; Baldys and Aust 2005).

Following the suggestion that the high iron content of crocidolite asbestos might explain its greater carcinogenicity when compared to chrysolite asbestos (Weinberg 1989), Dr. Ann Aust at Utah State University initiated a series of studies designed to unravel the role of iron and oxygen radicals in asbestos carcinogenicity. The studies of Dr. Aust and her various collaborators are unique and of incomparable value, as they are among the earliest studies regarding the role of iron in asbestos carcinogenicity, and have been continued for more than 15 years. A brief review follows:

- **1990**: Lund and Aust studied mobilization of iron from crocidolite by ascorbic acid and iron chelators: "These results suggest that iron can be mobilized from asbestos in the cell by low-molecular-weight chelators. If this occurs, it may have deleterious effects because this could result in deregulation of normal iron metabolism by proteins within the cell, resulting in iron-catalyzed oxidation of biomolecules."
- **1991a, 1991b**: Lund and Aust extended the studies on iron as the carcinogenic factor in asbestos by using iron chelators, demonstrating that a variety of chelators make the iron more redox active which results in greater oxygen consumption and increased production of oxygen radicals.
- **1992**: Lund and Aust reported that iron associated with asbestos catalyzes damage to DNA. "...the results of the present study strongly suggest that iron was responsible for asbestos-dependent generation of oxygen radicals, which resulted in the formation of DNA single-strand breaks."
- **1994**: Lund et al. extended previous studies by isolating amosite corded asbestos bodies from human lungs. When asbestos enters the human lung, a coat material is deposited

on the fibers, apparently in an effort by the lung defenses to isolate the fiber from the lung surface. Iron is then deposited on the asbestos fibers, which increases the damage to biomolecules above that of the uncoated fibers.

- **1995**: Hardy and Aust demonstrated that fibers such as crocidolite may be able to bind iron from intracellular sources. "This additional iron may be as reactive as the intrinsic iron and may increase reactive lifetime of the fiber."

- **1996**: Chao et al. demonstrated that human lung carcinoma cells can mobilize iron from crocidolite. This interesting study employed neutron-activated crocidolite, which contained iron isotopes. The neutron-activated crocidolite was then phagocytized by human lung carcinoma cells. Release of iron from phagocytized crocidolite resulted in iron overload and decreased cell survival.

- **1997**: Fang and Aust demonstrated the induction of ferritin synthesis in human lung epithelial cells in response to crocidolite asbestos. Ferritin is the protein molecule that sequesters excess iron, thereby preventing redox cycling and oxidative damage. Apparently, human lung cells attempt to protect themselves from iron contained in asbestos, but that protection is not always adequate.

- **1998a**: Park and Aust employed an ingenious method in an attempt to unravel the role of oxygen radicals in DNA damage induced by crocidolite asbestos. Others had previously demonstrated that some sections of DNA are susceptible to oxidative damage, whereas other portions are not. Crocidolite asbestos induced mutation in the oxidation-sensitive center, but not in the oxidation-stable region, indicating, once more, that crocidolite toxicity to DNA is due to generation of oxygen radicals.

- **1998b**: Park and Aust—"Treatment of human lung epithelial (A549) cells with crocidolite asbestos resulted in the induction of the inducible form of nitric oxide synthase, production of nitric oxide, and a dramatic decrease in intracellular reduced glutathione." Glutathione is a reducing agent produced by cells as a defense against oxidative damage. Nitric oxide may be further oxidized by iron, producing a damaging oxygen radical, peroxynitrite.

- **2000**: Shen et al. described a method for depositing iron on asbestos fibers in vitro in order to develop further studies that may help to unravel the mechanism by which iron induces DNA damage.
- **2005**: Baldys and Aust examined two plausible mechanisms by which asbestos exerts its pathologic effects: 1) Asbestos-induced pulmonary toxicity might be initiated by reactive oxygen species generated by redox cycling of iron; 2) Asbestos fibers may interact with the cellular membrane, causing changes in signaling mechanisms that are involved in cancer development. Others had already demonstrated that one of the signaling mechanisms affected in rodent cells involves the receptor protein for epidermal growth factor, leading to cell death (apoptosis). This study extended earlier studies to human lung cells, human pleural mesothelial cells, and normal human small airway epithelial cells. This effect was directly related to the amount of iron mobilized from the fibers.

The mechanisms by which asbestos causes cancer are still not completely known, but continuing research in Dr. Aust's laboratory—and in many other laboratories throughout the world—demonstrate beyond reasonable doubt that iron is involved in asbestos carcinogenicity. Asbestos-iron, similar to iron-dextran and possibly iron gluconate, is an established human carcinogen.

Iron in Cigarette Smoke and Fly Ash

Polycyclic aromatic hydrocarbons (PAHs) are important procarcinogens in cigarette smoke. The term, "procarcinogens," means that the PAHs are not directly carcinogenic, but must first be converted to their carcinogenic forms. The major activation pathway for PAHs is through oxidation catalyzed by a group of enzymes known as cytochromes P450. Cytochromes P450 use iron to catalyze the oxidation of most xenobiotics ("foreign compounds"). Most of the "tar" in tobacco smoke is acted on by cytochromes P450 (reviewed in Xue and Warshawsky 2005).

This oxidation by cytochromes P450 results in substances known as PAH-diol-epoxides. Iron can, by itself, oxidize PAHs through a Fenton-driven reaction (Nadarajah et al. 2002; Garcon et al. 2004a, 2004b). That is apparently what happens in scrotal cancer and lung cancer induced by PAHs—the iron in inhaled cigarette smoke, or in soot smeared over the scrotum, activates PAHs. The PAH-diol-epoxides may themselves be carcinogenic. However, the current concept is that these partially oxidized PAHs are further activated to their PAH-ortho-quinone derivatives, which are the proximate carcinogenic metabolites (Shimada 2006; Cavalieri et al. 2005; Shimada and Fujii-Kuriyama 2004; Mimura and Fujii-Kuriyama 2003). The PAH-diol-epoxides or the PAH-ortho-quinones attach directly to DNA (Baird et al. 2005; Randernath et al. 1992), where they are available for redox cycling using iron as a catalyst. The redox cycling of the PAH-diol-epoxides and/or the PAH-ortho-quinones damages the DNA, thereby initiating carcinogenesis.

Sources of inhaled iron that may result in respiratory cancers include: 1) fly ash emitted from burning coal or wood; 2) volatile tars in cigarette smoke; 3) inhaled asbestos; and 4) industrial exposure among miners and steel workers. There is substantial evidence that oxygen radical generation induced by redox cycling of iron is involved in these cancers (van Maanen et al. 1999; Smith et al. 2000; Ball et al. 2000; Weinberg 1981, 1989, 1992a, 1993, 1996a, 2001).

Iron and Scrotal Cancer

The story of scrotal cancer among chimney sweeps takes us back in time to early industrial England. During 1600s-1700s, coal or wood was used as fuel, and fireplaces had chimneys that were larger than our chimneys are today. Their chimneys were large enough for the men who were chimney sweeps to climb upward through them (or pass downward through them) while performing the chore of cleaning the chimney. They wore minimal or no clothing. Thus, there was a high incidence of scrotal cancer among chimney sweeps. It has been known since that time that soot from burning things is carcinogenic. However, the reason for the carcinogenicity of soot or cigarette smoke was unknown until quite recently, and only at the present time is more complete information becoming available (Shimada 2006; Cavalieri et al. 2005; Shimada and Fujii-Kuriyama 2004).

Increased Liver Iron: Hepatocellular Carcinoma

> *"The liver is a principal target for iron toxicity because it is chiefly responsible for taking up and storing excessive amounts of iron."* (Bonkovsky and Lambrecht 2000.)

In the following discussion, evidence will be summarized that dietary iron acts directly to cause liver cancer. As well, iron is a co-carcinogen, with all other risk factors for hepatocellular carcinoma: 1) hepatitis B and C infections; 2) aflatoxin-contaminated food; 3) alcohol; 4) tobacco use; and 5) other chemical carcinogens.

> Hepatocellular cancer is the fifth most frequent cancer in men and the eighth in women worldwide. Established risk factors are chronic hepatitis B and C infection, chronic heavy alcohol consumption, obesity and type 2 diabetes, tobacco use, use of oral contraceptives, and aflatoxin-contaminated food. Almost 90% of all hepatocellular carcinomas develop in cirrhotic livers. In Western countries, attributable risks are highest for cirrhosis due to chronic alcohol abuse and viral hepatitis B and C infection.... An important mechanism implicated in alcohol-related hepatocarcinogenesis is oxidative stress from alcohol metabolism, inflammation, and increased iron storage. (Seitz and Stickel 2006)

That iron overload is associated with a high risk for hepatic carcinogenesis was summarized by Huang (2003). This is illustrated by the fact that a common complication of hereditary hemochromatosis is the development of hepatocellular carcinoma, which affects approximately 30% of patients with pathological iron deposition in parenchymal tissue (Deugnier and Turlin 2001; Turlin and Deugnier 2002; Huang 2003; Deugnier 2003; Peterson 2005; Deugnier and Turlin 2007). It is believed that iron overload disrupts the redox balance of the cell and generates chronic oxidative stress, which modulates signaling networks related to malignant transformation (Benhar et al. 2002).

Dietary iron overload occurs commonly in parts of sub-Saharan Africa as a result of consumption of large volumes of traditional beer that is home-brewed in iron pots. Although dietary iron overload was not originally believed to cause hepatocellular carcinoma, recent case-control studies have shown that African Blacks with dietary iron overload are, indeed, at increased risk for hepatocellular carcinoma (Kew and Asare 2007).

Dietary Iron Overload

> *"Our findings are compatible with the hypothesis that the direct hepatocarcinogenic effect of free iron is mediated by the generation of oxygen reactive species and oxidative damage that are mutagenic and carcinogenic."*
>
> (Asare et al. 2006a)

Ordinarily in human hepatocellular carcinomas, cirrhosis precedes the development of cancerous cells. For this reason, until recently, it has not been possible to determine if iron excess is directly carcinogenic, even though the mutagenicity of various types of iron has been clearly demonstrated (Sahu and Washington 1991; Dunkel et al. 1999). A number of animal models have been developed in an attempt to determine if iron is directly carcinogenic.

Sahu and Washington (1991) demonstrated iron-mediated oxidative DNA damage in isolated rat liver nuclei. Kang et al. (1998) developed a rat model for assessment of iron overload in hemochromatosis; however, hepatocellular carcinoma did not develop in these rats. Pigeon et al. (1999) fed a strain of male mice varying amounts of supplements of iron-carbonyl for varying periods of time from 2 to 12 months. The mice receiving high levels of iron-carbonyl developed significant iron overload and nuclear changes in hepatocytes; however, they did not develop liver fibrosis or hepatocellular carcinoma after 12 months. Masini et al. (2000) demonstrated irreversible mitochondrial dysfunction and fibrosis in the liver of chronic iron-dosed gerbils; however, hepatocellular carcinoma did not develop. Thus, as the 20th century came to an end, the question whether iron is directly hepatocarcinogenic had not been resolved.

Even though it was not possible to demonstrate direct carcinogenicity for iron in these early animal models, the hepatotoxicity of iron overload resulting in fibrosis, cirrhosis, and liver cancer continued to be a subject for regular editorials and reviews (Britton et al. 1987; Bacon and Britton 1989; Bonkovsky 1991; Bacon et al. 1993; Britton.et al. 1994; Britton and Bacon 1994; Stål 1995; Britton 1996; Abalea et al. 1998; Olynyk 1999; Bonkovsky and Lambrecht 2000; Huang 2003; Pietrangelo 2002; Pietrangelo 2003; Peterson 2005; Seitz and Stickel 2006;Valko et al. 2006).

Asare and collaborators have recently developed the necessary animal model that demonstrates quite clearly that dietary iron carbonyl (a form of iron approved by the FDA for addition to food) is directly carcinogenic (Asare et al. 2006a, 2006b). Male Wistar rats fed varying levels of iron carbonyl developed hepatocellular carcinoma in the absence of liver fibrosis. Asare et al. (2006b) state, "We conclude that hepatocellular carcinoma may complicate dietary hepatic iron overload in Wistar albino rats in the absence of fibrosis or cirrhosis, confirming an aetiological association between dietary iron overload and the tumor and suggesting that iron may be directly hepatocarcinogenic."

Iron is a Co-carcinogen with Hepatitis B and C Viral Infections

"Long-term iron depletion for chronic hepatitis C patients is a promising modality for lowering the risk of progression to hepatocellular carcinoma." (Kato et al. 2007)

Several viruses have a high affinity for the liver, where they cause inflammation, cirrhosis, and liver cancer. Of these, the two most important are the hepatitis B and C viruses. An estimated 1.25 million Americans are chronically infected with the hepatitis B virus, and around 3.2 million are chronically infected with hepatitis C.

A relation between increased liver iron and other abnormal parameters of iron metabolism in chronic hepatitis B infection has been known for more than 30 years (Sutknik et al. 1974; reviewed by Bacon 1997). Blumberg and colleagues (Sutknik et al. 1974) described abnormal iron status in patients with hepatitis B infection, and Prieto and colleagues (1975) reported iron overload in chronic and acute liver disease. Since that time, numerous studies have confirmed abnormal iron metabolism frequently leading to hepatocellular carcinoma in hepatitis B and C infections and in alcoholic liver disease. In an animal model using transgenic mice expressing the hepatitis C virus polyprotein, hepatic iron overload has been demonstrated to result in hepatocellular carcinoma (Furutani et al. 2006). Nishina et al. (2008) demonstrated that hepatitis C virus raises hepatic iron level in mice by reducing production of hepcidin.

An analysis of the third National Health and Nutrition Examination Survey (NHANES III) showed that hepatitis C infection is significantly associated with higher serum levels of ferritin and iron in the U.S. population (Shan et al. 2005). Previous NHANES reports also indicated a subpopulation with elevated iron parameters. Unfortunately, the Food and Nutrition Board (1993) chose to ignore this group, concentrating only on the "iron-deficient" population in keeping with its predetermined goal to defeat iron deficiency at all cost.

Very few drugs are available for treatment of viral liver infections. Only two have been commonly used. Interferons are a group of polypeptides produced by certain cells in response to viral infection—once produced the interferon binds to the surface of uninfected cells, stimulating them to synthesize antiviral proteins that block viral replication. The response to interferon therapy is dependent on liver iron stores—the higher the iron content of the liver, the less likely a patient will respond to interferon therapy (Van

Thiel et al. 1994; Olynyk et al. 1995; Barton et al. 1995; Piperano et al. 1996; Fargion et al. 1997).

Ribavirin is a more recently developed antiviral drug. Similar to the circumstance with interferon therapy, the outcome of hepatic viral infection treated with ribavirin is adversely affected by elevated liver iron stores (Distante et al. 2002; Fujita et al. 2007a, 2007b).

A common contemporary approach to treating hepatitis C infection is iron depletion via low-iron diet therapy and/or phlebotomy. Alexander et al. (2007) performed weekly phlebotomies on eighteen patients with chronic hepatitis C infection who did not respond to interferon therapy. Phlebotomy was continued until iron depletion was confirmed by serum ferritin less than 50 ng/ml. "Iron depletion was associated with a biochemical response in 22% of patients who did not respond to interferon monotherapy. There was a significant reduction in a key marker of fibrogenesis among patients with biochemical response. These data support longer-term studies of iron depletion in chronic hepatitis C."

Sumida et al. (2007) compared dietary iron reduction with phlebotomy in treating patients with chronic hepatitis C infection and found phlebotomy superior to dietary iron reduction. Kato et al. (2007) combined long-term phlebotomy with low-iron diet. "Long-term iron depletion for chronic hepatitis C patients is a promising modality for lowering the risk of progression to hepatocellular carcinoma."

Although hereditary hemochromatosis is a well-known risk factor for liver cancer, an intensive search for other hereditary risk factors has not yet proven successful (reviewed in Valenti et al. 2007). Understanding the role of iron dysmetabolism in hepatitis B and C infection and in alcoholic liver disease is the most crucial factor that will lead to understanding and treating these diseases (Oates and West 2006).

Hepatic Iron Overload and Alcoholic Liver Disease

"...increased hepatic iron content is associated with greater mortality from alcoholic cirrhosis, suggesting

a pathogenic role for iron in alcoholic liver disease....
Alcohol and iron appear to act synergistically to cause
liver injury."   (Harrison-Findik 2007)

The relationship between alcohol, iron, and oxidative liver damage is very complex—far beyond the scope of the present limited review. Comprehensive reviews have been published. Two of the most extensive are those of Cederbaum (1992) and Dey and Cederbaum (2006). The review by Dey and Cederbaum (2006) is of exceptional importance as it appeared in the 25th Anniversary Issue of *Hepatology*, a journal that has published many of the seminal reports on this topic.

In addition, the proceedings of a recent symposium on the role of iron in alcoholic liver disease is found in *Alcohol* 30, No. 2, 2003. All articles in that symposium confirm a role for iron in hepatotoxicity of alcohol (Brittenham 2003; Deugnier 2003; Bonkovsky et al. 2003; Fletcher and Powell 2003; Pietrangelo 2003; Cederbaum 2003; Xiong et al. 2003; Rouault 2003; Swanson 2003; Purohit et al. 2003).

DeFeo et al. (2001) reported an increase in non-transferrin-bound iron in alcohol abusers, which they suggested may have a role in initiating or promoting alcohol-induced liver damage. Suzuki et al. (2002) found an increase in transferrin receptors in hepatocytes from habitual alcohol users indicating that habitual alcohol drinking results in an increase in transferrin receptors with consequent hepatic iron overload in alcoholic liver disease. Fletcher et al. (2003) reviewed the role of consumption of excess alcohol in patients with liver iron storage diseases, in particular in hereditary hemochromatosis, where co-existent alcohol and iron are implicated in end-stage liver disease. Ioannou et al. (2007) found elevated serum transferrin-iron saturation resulting from excessive alcohol consumption, suggesting that iron overload and alcohol act in synergy to promote hepatic fibrogenesis and carcinogenesis.

Because there is no physiologic method for excreting iron, iron homeostasis is largely controlled by iron absorption. As previously discussed, hepcidin is a protein produced in the liver that decreases iron absorption. A diet containing elevated levels of iron results in an increase in hepcidin synthesis in the liver, which results in decreased iron absorption. This mechanism holds true for humans, rats, and mice, and protects from iron overload on high iron ingestion. The more iron in the diet, the greater the hepcidin synthesis, which reduces the amount of iron absorbed. Alcohol decreases hepcidin synthesis, and increases the level of iron transporter in the intestine, resulting in increased iron absorption even in the presence of adequate iron stores (Harrison-Findik et al. 2006, 2007).

Iron Overload and Aflatoxins

Aflatoxins are carcinogenic compounds produced by many species of *Aspergillus* fungi. Exposure to a combination of aflatoxin B_1 and iron overload are important causes of hepatocellular carcinoma in sub-Saharan Africa. Asare et al. (2007) investigated the possible interaction of the two risk factors in Wistar albino rats. When combined, these two risk factors demonstrated a multiplicative effect of around five-fold on the end-points of mutagenesis.

Shen et al. (1995) studied the involvement of reactive oxygen species in aflatoxin-B_1-induced cell injury in rat hepatocytes. Addition of oxygen radical scavengers (superoxide dismutase, catalase, or dimethyl sulfoxide), or the iron chelator, desferrioxamine, inhibited damage produced by aflatoxin B_1. The authors conclude that generation of reactive oxygen species generated by redox cycling of iron is involved in aflatoxin B_1 cell injury in cultured rat hepatocytes.

High Iron Stores Sensitize to Ionizing Radiation
"These results indicate that a sublethal concentration of ferritin can be a potent radiosensitiser." (Stevens 1992)

Exposure of human populations to high-energy radiation, whether from occupational, medical, or environmental sources, may result in radiation injury such as cataracts, skin aging, damage to biomembranes, and DNA damage leading to cancer. There is general population awareness that ionizing radiation [short ultraviolet rays from the sun (UVA), X-rays, and gamma-rays] can cause cancer. Consequently, sunscreens that block much of the UVA are now widely used. However, few people know that ionizing radiation exerts its damaging effects by a mechanism that involves iron-catalyzed active oxygen species. It is the hydroxyl radical ($\cdot$OH) that causes most of the damage.

As a result of this newer knowledge, a new generation of sunscreens is now evolving. These sunscreens incorporate an iron-chelating agent in the UVA blocking cream, and are proven to be far more effective than sun blockers alone. Since the skin-aging effects of sunshine are generated by a mechanism that requires iron, it will not be long before the cosmetic industry will begin incorporating iron chelators into cosmetic skin creams.

Iron Increases the Damaging Effects of Ionizing Radiation

This story begins in 1981 when Kong et al. reported the damaging effects of gamma-radiation on erythrocyte ghosts, and Kong and Davison (1981) demonstrated that the damaging effects of gamma-radiation are mediated by the hydroxyl radical ($\cdot$OH). Repine et al. (1981) showed that the hydroxyl radical scavenger, dimethyl sulfoxide, prevented 80% of the single-strand breaks in isolated DNA, and 100% of the single-strand breaks induced by an iron/hydrogen peroxide system. This led to the conclusion that 80% of the DNA damage caused by gamma rays is due to the hydroxyl radical. In the same year, Stitch and collaborators (Whiting et al. 1981) demonstrated that ferritin (a source of iron) can have damaging effects on chromosomes, which are prevented by an iron chelator. Epidemiological studies supported the hypothesis that increased body iron stores increase the risk of cancer (Stevens 1990; Stevens et al. 1988; Selby and Friedman 1988).

However, the relationship between gamma-radiation, iron, and chromosome damage remained relatively unexplored for nearly a decade when Nelson and Stevens (1991) became the first to demonstrate that ferritin-iron sensitizes mammalian cells to radiation-induced damage. From these studies, Stevens et al. (2000) conclude: "Chronically increased oxidative stress from elevated levels of iron in the body may increase radiation sensitivity by decreasing cellular oxygen radical scavenging capability. Hemochromatosis heterozygotes have elevated body iron. Low-level radiation sensitization by iron may be particularly pertinent for the risk of breast cancer. Since 10% of the population appears to be heterozygous for the hemochromatosis gene, a radiosensitizing effect would have pervasive implications."

Since 1991, Tyrrell & Pouzard and their various collaborators have reported detailed studies on the mechanisms by which ionizing radiation, iron, and the hydroxyl radical activate oxidative stress signals (Tyrrell 1991, 1996; Vile et al. 1995; Vile and Tyrrell 1995; Pouzard and Tyrrell 1999; Pouzard et al. 1999a, 1999b; Kvam et al. 2000; Reelfs et al. 2004; Zhong et al. 2004). Avunduk et al. (2000) demonstrated that x-ray exposure causes toxic cell injury in the rat lens by releasing iron that catalyzes hydroxyl radical generation.

Caged-Iron Chelators in Sunscreens and Cosmetics

Bissett et al. (1991) and Bissett and McBride (1996) emphasized the importance of topical iron chelators to protect skin cells against the UV-induced increase in skin iron. Strong iron chelators such as desferrioxamine mesylate (DFO) suppress both cell damage (Zhong et al. 2004) and iron release (Pouzard et al. 1999; Kvam et al. 2000; Reelfs et al. 2004; Zhong et al. 2004). Unfortunately, prolonged dosing with exposure to strong iron chelators leads to side effects as a result of the removal of essential iron from various sites including iron-containing enzymes (Porter and Huens 1989; Singh et al. 1995; Hileti et al. 1995; Rakba et al. 2000; Simonart et al. 2002).

To minimize these side effects, a series of photoprotective iron-chelation strategies have been proposed in oxidative conditions (Galey et al. 2000; Séité et al. 2004). Yu et al. (2003) utilized amifostine, an inorganic triphosphate that requires dephosphorylation to produce the active radioprotective agent. Amifostine is used clinically to minimize damage from radiation therapy to adjacent normal tissues. Alternatively, design of a mild iron chelator [N-(4-pyridoxylmethylene)-1-serine (PYSer)] derived from serine and vitamin B6 (Kitazawa et al. 2005) has been reported to considerably reduce the observed toxic side effects by strong iron chelators.

The most significant advance in the attempt to develop non-damaging iron chelators that can be used for photoprotection has been developed by Yiakouvaki et al. (2006). These iron chelators are referred to as a "caged-iron chelators." They involve a strong iron chelator that is attached to a chemical structure that prevents their iron chelating ability. However, on exposure to radiation, the chemical structure that prevents iron chelation (the 'caging' agent) is removed, and the iron chelator is released. At least two variations of "caged-iron chelators" have been developed and are being tested on skin cells (Yiakouvaki et al. 2006).

Lactoferrin or Ovotransferrin in Sunscreens and Cosmetics

Lactoferrin is the iron-binding glycoprotein secreted in milk, lachrymal glands, and other body secretions. Lactoferrin has antibiotic and anti-cancer properties (Weinberg 1996, 2002, 2005, 2007). Since lactoferrin is a natural secretion and does not damage sensitive tissues such as eyes and breasts, and since it has powerful iron-binding qualities, lactoferrin may soon find its way into sunscreens and cosmetics.

Ovotransferrin (ovalbumin) has iron-binding qualities similar to lactoferrin and might be preferred since it is far less expensive. Lactoferrin is currently produced by recombinant DNA procedures whereas egg white is the readily available source of ovotransferrin. Egg white has been used to beautify the skin—perhaps science has uncovered the reason for this!

Increased Iron Stores are Associated with Breast Cancer

Epidemiological studies have suggested an association between consuming red meat and the development of several kinds of cancer, including breast cancer. It has been suggested that heme iron is involved. A few studies have not confirmed this observation. That is the nature of epidemiology—it is not an exact science. Epidemiology can point the way to help in the discovery of cause of disease, but cannot provide proof of a causal relationship.

Clinical and experimental studies are needed to prove or disprove hypotheses generated by epidemiological studies. Some of the evidence that strongly suggests that high iron stores are closely associated with breast cancer includes: 1) Hemochromatosis gene mutations associated with increased iron absorption predispose to breast cancer; 2) Increased serum ferritin is found in patients with breast cancer; 3) Abnormal ferritin-bearing lymphocytes are found in women with breast cancer; 4) Increased iron levels are found in women with malignant breast cancer as compared with benign cases; and 5) Estrogen, used to induce cancer in laboratory animals, increases body accumulation of iron.

Epidemiology Regarding Iron and Breast Cancer

The epidemiology regarding the role of dietary heme iron in breast cancer is contradictory. Recent studies include:

- A Chinese study of serum markers in breast cancer mortality (Guo et al. 1994), which analyzed data from 65 Chinese rural counties. Analysis indicated that "consumption of animal foods, including eggs, fish, and meat was positively linked to country-wide mortality rates of breast cancer in Chinese women." And "Positive correlations for serum ferritin and hemoglobin were found."
- The Shanghai Breast Cancer Study (Kallianpur et al. 2007, 2008). The authors investigated the effects of iron and fats from various food sources on the risk of breast cancer in a population-based case-control study involving 3,452 breast cancer cases compared to 3,474 age-frequency-matched controls, and concluded, "A high intake of animal-derived (heme) iron may be associated with an increased risk of primary breast cancer in Chinese women, and saturated and

mono-unsaturated fats that are also derived from animal sources may augment this effect. Combined reductions in animal-derived iron and fat consumption have the potential to reduce breast cancer risk."

- A Canadian study of heme iron intake and the risk of breast cancer "found no association of iron or heme iron intake with breast cancer risk or for a modification by iron of the effect of alcohol or estrogen." (Kabat et al. 2007.) This study involved 49,654 women ages 40 to 59 followed for an average of 16.4 years. Two thousand five hundred and forty five (2,545) incident breast cancer cases were identified. From this, Kabat and Rohan (2007) concluded that the hypothesis that excess iron plays a role in breast carcinogenesis remains unresolved.

There have been many other studies of the relationship between dietary red meat and breast cancer. A full review is beyond the scope of this book. For now, it is sufficient to state that the epidemiology relating to consumption of red meat and breast cancer has provided contradictory results, although most studies have reported that consumption of red meat is positively correlated with breast cancer development. Because epidemiology has not provided answers, we must examine the rest of the information in order to help resolve the relationship between high iron stores and breast cancer.

HFE Gene Mutations and Breast Cancer

Kallianpur et al. (2004) studied the prevalence of a hemochromatosis mutation (*HFE C282Y*) in women with breast cancer. Individuals with the *C282Y* hemochromatosis allele and iron overload are known to develop hepatocellular carcinoma and some extrahepatic malignancies at increased rates. However, previous studies had not reported on *C282Y* allele in relation to breast cancer. Because 1 in 10 Caucasians of Northern European ancestry carries this allele, any impact it may have on breast cancer burden is potentially great. The authors state, "We report a high prevalence of *C282Y* alleles in a cohort of breast cancer patients who underwent high-dose chemotherapy and blood cell transplantation (BCT) for poor-prognosis disease. An increased prevalence of this allele, although less pronounced, was observed in a nontransplant sample of women with primary invasive breast cancer. These findings suggest a possible link between altered iron metabolism in *C282Y* carriers and the pathophysiology of breast cancer."

Gunel-Ozcan et al. (2006) studied the occurrence of another hemochromatosis mutation (*HFE H63D*) frequency in Turkish women with breast cancer. The study indicated that women with the H63D mutation had more than twice the risk. The authors conclude, "Our results suggest that *HFE H63D* mutation frequencies were increased in breast cancer patients compared to those in the general population. Also, odds ratios (odds ratio = 2.05) computed in this study suggest that *H63D* has a positive association with breast cancer."

Oxidative Stress and Breast Cancer

Hong et al. (2007) reported a nested case-control study of postmenopausal women (505 cases and 502 cohorts) from the American Cancer Society Prevention II Nutrition Cohort. They examined the relationships between breast cancer risk and genetic polymorphisms of enzymes involved in the generation and removal of iron-mediated reactive oxygen species and concluded, "These results indicate that women with genotypes resulting in potentially higher levels of iron-generated oxidative stress may be at increased risk of breast cancer and that this association may be most relevant among women with high iron intake."

Increased Levels of Serum Ferritin in Breast Cancer

The most important measurements to determine a person's iron status are serum ferritin and transferrin loading. Normal serum ferritin is 25-50 ng/mL (nanograms per milliliter), and transferrin loading is 30-35%. Elevated levels of either value indicate excess circulating iron or iron storage. Elevated serum ferritin is generally found in patients with breast cancer. Because different laboratories may report differing levels of serum ferritin, in the following discussion the values given have been recorded as they appear in the articles. The author's statements that the levels are elevated have been recorded as stated in the article.

In an early study before serum ferritin measurements became standardized, Marcus and Zinberg (1975) used a double-antibody radioimmunoassay for measurement of serum ferritin. Using this assay, they defined an upper limit of normal as 146 ng/ml for women (mean 34 ng/ml). Serum ferritin levels exceeded this in preoperative sera of 41% of women with mammary carcinoma (mean 199 ng/ml) and in 67% of women with locally recurrent or metastatic mammary carcinoma (mean 671 ng/ml). The authors suggested that "measurement of serum ferritin may be useful in evaluation of patients with breast cancer and in monitoring their response to therapy."

Ulbrich et al. (2003) designed a study to determine the incidence of anemia in patients with breast cancer (n=84), ductal carcinoma in situ (n=29) fibroadenoma (n=100), and healthy women (n=14). Their results indicated, "Serum ferritin was significantly elevated in breast cancer. Among patients with breast cancer, a significant correlation with positive lymph node involvement was noted. Elevated serum ferritin might indicate the presence of malignant disease and could be regarded as a predictor of positive lymph node involvement in patients with breast cancer."

High Ferritin Concentrations and Recurrence of Breast Cancer

Jacobs et al. (1976) studied serum ferritin concentration in early breast cancer. They measured circulating ferritin in 250 normal adult women and 229 women presenting with early breast cancer. Ferritin concentrations were found to be higher in the breast cancer patients than in normal women, and, "Patients with an initial circulating ferritin concentration above 200 mìg/l have a higher tumor recurrence rate during the subsequent 4 years."

Weinstein et al. (1989) reported a seven-year follow-up study on 36 breast cancer patients in whom breast tissue ferritin concentrations at the time of surgery were known. Of these, 86% of patients with low tissue ferritin survived free of recurrence or second tumor versus 40% with high tissue ferritin concentrations. This suggests that increased tissue ferritin increases recurrence of breast cancer.

Elevated Iron in Benign Breast Tissue

Cui et al. (2007) conducted a case-control study involving 252 matched pairs nested in a cohort of 9,315 women with benign breast disease. Levels of zinc, selenium, calcium, and iron were measured in breast tissue from these subjects. "In conclusion, our data raise the possibility that relatively high levels of zinc, iron, and calcium in benign breast tissue may be associated with a modest increased risk of subsequent breast cancer.

Abnormal Ferritin-Bearing Lymphocytes

Among the most interesting findings in breast cancer patients is the occurrence of abnormal ferritin-bearing T-lymphocytes in breast cancer patients (Giler and Moroz 1978; Moroz et al. 1984; Papenhausen et al. 1984; Pattanapanyasat et al. 1988; Rosen et al. 1992, 1992a, 1992b, 1992c). Giler and Moroz (1978) were first to report this interesting phenomenon: "Recently a subpopulation of circulating T lymphocytes bearing surface ferritin was found in patients with breast cancer and untreated Hodgkin's disease. No such lymphocytes were demonstrated in normals or in patients with benign breast disease. The appearance of such a subpopulation in the circulation is an early manifestation of neoplastic disease, and its identification may provide a tool of potential diagnostic and prognostic importance in the management of Hodgkin's disease and breast cancer." The significance of this discovery still remains unknown, but it is a definite indication of abnormal iron metabolism in breast cancer patients.

Iron and Estrogens

Most major risk factors for breast cancer are hormonal or reproductive factors that increase exposure to estrogen and/or progesterone (Pike et al. 1993), and its effects are mediated primarily through the estrogen receptors, termed alpha and beta (Conway et al. 2007). Estrogens exert a proliferative effect on breast cells, and anti-estrogens have been used to inhibit or reverse neoplastic progression of breast cells to clinical breast cancer (Cyrus-Davis and Strom 2001). In areas such as Marin County, California, an exceptionally high incidence of breast cancer is correlated with estrogen receptor positive breast cancer cells (Benz et al. 2003). The risk of hormone dependent breast cancer increases with aging (Vrbanec and Petriceviæ 2007). It is, therefore, important to examine the relationship, if any, between iron and estrogen in breast cancer development.

There has been little interest in the association of iron with estrogen in breast cancer development. A study from Japan is the first to demonstrate the elevation of serum iron level with oral administration of medoxyprogesterone acetate in patients with breast cancer (Kadota et al. 1991).

Wyllie and Liehr (1997) demonstrated that redox cycling of estrogen metabolites releases iron(II) from ferritin, which in turn generates hydroxyl radicals by a Fenton reaction, and suggested that redox cycling of iron with estrogen contributes to tumor initiation in breast cells. Subsequently, Wyllie and Liehr (1998) showed that dietary iron enhances estrogen-induced renal tumors in hamsters. Liehr and Jones (2001) demonstrated that elevated dietary iron increases estrogen-induced breast cancer in rats. As well, estrogen administration increases iron accumulation in hamsters and facilitates iron uptake by cells in culture (Liehr and Jones 2001). Liehr and Jones (2001) conclude, "A role of iron in hormone-associated cancer in humans offers attractive routes for cancer prevention by regulating metal ion metabolism and interfering with iron accumulation in tissues."

Dai et al. (2007) demonstrated that the estrogens and iron act synergistically to increase cell proliferations in estrogen receptor positive cancer cells.

Iron and Colon Cancer

As we embark on a discussion of the role of iron in colon cancer, it might be well to keep in mind the proposed role for iron in various forms of cancer that we have reviewed. In the cases of injected iron and inhaled iron, iron's carcinogenicity is independent of the body iron stores. No matter what a person's iron status may be, the inhaled or injected iron is available to induce cancer.

In liver, skin, and breast cancer, excessive levels of iron are found. Of course, once any form of cancer has developed, body iron stores may be depleted because cancer cells preferentially acquire iron. The association between the progression stage of cancer and anemia is well known and will be discussed later.

In contrast to liver, skin, and breast cancer, colon cancer is associated with anemia and depleted body iron stores. A bit of thought will reveal that this might be anticipated because colon cancer is associated with dietary iron that has not been absorbed. It is the iron that enters the colon, not the iron that is absorbed, that is important. In fact, the information we are about to consider suggests that people who develop colon cancer may very well be those who, for whatever reason, are unable to absorb enough iron from ingested food, which results in more iron passing into the colon. Clearly, treatment of the anemia associated with colon cancer by iron supplementation may be dangerous. Treating anemia in cancer patients by giving blood transfusions is associated with increased infection risk, tumor recurrence, and mortality (Dunne et al. 2002).

Reduced Iron Levels in Colorectal Cancer

Because consuming red meat rich in heme iron is associated with colon cancer risk, a number of researchers have determined the iron status of people with colon cancer. Most of these studies have found low or normal iron stores as measured by serum ferritin, transferrin saturation, and serum iron.

Kato et al. (1999) examined the relationship between iron status and colorectal cancer in a case-control study nested within the New York University Women's Health Study cohort. For 105 cases of colorectal cancer with an average follow-up of 4.7 years and 523 individually matched controls, baseline levels of serum iron, ferritin, total iron binding capacity, and transferrin saturation were determined as indicators. Serum ferritin was inversely associated with colon cancer incidence; the other measurements show no significant difference. However, an increased risk of colorectal cancer was associated with higher total iron intake among subjects with higher fat intake. This, they suggested, might be due to increased iron in the intestine which, combined with a high fat intake, may increase the risk of colon cancer.

Gackowski et al. (2002) compared serum iron and ferritin, transferrin saturation, and total iron binding capacity in 45 colorectal cancer patients and 51 healthy controls. Patients with colorectal cancer showed significantly lower values of transferrin saturation, total iron binding capacity and serum iron levels than controls.

Kucharzewski et al. (2003) compared serum iron levels in 67 patients with colorectal cancer and 42 patients with rectal polyps. Patients with colorectal cancer had lower levels of serum iron than the patients with polyps or controls, suggesting that low serum iron may increase colorectal cancer risk.

Cross et al. (2006) determined that serum ferritin, serum iron, and transferrin saturation were all inversely associated with colon cancer risk. The study included 130 colorectal cancer cases and 260 controls—colorectal cancer patients had lower values for all of these measures of iron status.

Iron Deficiency Anemia is Common in Colon Cancer

Talley et al. (1989) studied the potential risk for colorectal cancer in patients with pernicious anemia (pernicious anemia is due to vitamin B_{12} deficiency). They studied 150 residents of Rochester, Minnesota, who had the onset of pernicious anemia during the 30-year period from 1950-1970. The observed risk for colorectal cancer in these subjects was compared with that expected based on incidence rates of colon and rectal cancer for the local population. Although the overall risk was not significant, their data suggested that patients with pernicious anemia may have an increased risk for colorectal cancer in the 5 years after diagnosis.

Dunne et al. (2002) studied preoperative anemia in colon cancer patients. Data were collected on 311 patients diagnosed with colorectal cancer over a 6-year period from 1994 through 1999. Preoperative anemia was most common in patients with right colon cancer with an incidence of 57.6% followed by left colon cancer (42.2%) and rectal cancer (29.8%). The authors recommended complete colon evaluation in patients with anemia.

Raje et al. (2007) addressed the question, "What proportion of patients referred to secondary care with iron deficiency anemia have colon cancer?" They concluded that males referred with iron deficiency anemia have a significant risk of having colon cancer, whereas the risk seems lower in females.

Heme Iron and Colon Cancer

"Because iron is broadly supplemented in the American diet, the benefits of iron supplementation need to be measured against the long-term risks of increased iron exposure, one of which may be increased risk of colorectal cancer."　　　(Sinha 2004.)

"These data suggest that iron may confer an increased risk for colorectal cancer..."　　　(Wurzelman et al. 1996).

"...iron over-nutrition is proposed as a risk factor and dietary antioxidants as protective factors for ulcerative colitis-associated carcinogenesis."　　　(Seril et al. 2003.)

Many epidemiological studies have demonstrated that eating red meat is associated with colorectal cancer. Norat and Riboli (2001) reviewed the epidemiological evidence on colorectal cancer risk and meat consumption presented in 32 case-control and 13 cohort studies published in English from 1970 to 1999, concluding that consuming red meat and processed meat is associated with a moderate but significant increase in colorectal cancer risk. In a subsequent article, Norat et al. (2002) concluded that "the risk fraction attributable to current levels of red meat intake was in the range of 10-25% in regions where red meat intake is high. If average red meat intake is reduced to 70 g/week in these regions, colorectal cancer risk would hypothetically decrease by 7-24%." In 2005, Norat et al. (2005) published a study of 478,040 men and women from 10 European countries who were free of cancer at enrollment between 1992 and 1998. "In this study population, the absolute risk of development of colorectal cancer within 10 years for a study subject aged 50 years was 1.71% for the highest category of red and processed meat intake and 1.28% for subjects in the lowest category of intake...Our data confirm that colorectal cancer risk is positively associated with high consumption of red and processed meat..."

Wurzelmann et al. (1996) prospectively gathered data from the National Health and Nutrition Examination Survey I and the National Health Evaluation Follow-Up Study in order to evaluate the risk of colorectal cancer due to consumption of iron. Morbidity and mortality data due to colorectal cancer were available on 14,407 persons first interviewed in 1971 and followed through 1986. A total of 194 possible colorectal cancers occurred in this group over the 15-year period. The authors conclude, "These data suggest that iron may confer an increased risk for colorectal cancer, and that the localization of risk may be attributable to the mode of epithelial exposure. It seems that luminal exposure to iron increases risk proximally, whereas humoral exposure increases risk distally."

Seril et al. (2003) studied the relationship between chronic inflammatory bowel disease, ulcerative colitis, and colorectal cancer. Ulcerative colitis (UC) occurs commonly in the U.S. and Canada, but its etiology is unknown. An association between UC and an elevated risk for colorectal cancer is well established. The authors state, "The available evidence suggests that DNA damage caused by oxidative stress in the damage-regeneration cycle is a major contributor to colorectal cancer development in ulcerative colitis patients. Based on this concept, iron over-nutrition is proposed as a risk factor and dietary antioxidants as protective factors for ulcerative colitis and associated carcinogenesis."

Recent studies from Sweden, Australia, and the United States, confirm this association (Larsson et al. 2004, 2005a, 2005b). The Swedish Mammography Cohort Study (Larsson et al. 2004) concluded, "These findings suggest the high consumption of red meat may substantially increase the risk of distal colon cancer." A study from the Cancer Epidemiology Centre, Melbourne, Australia (English et al. 2004) concluded, "Consumption of fresh red meat and processed meat seemed to be associated with an increased risk of rectal cancer." A study conducted by the Epidemiology and Surveillance Research, American Cancer Society, Atlanta, Georgia (Chao et al. 2005) concluded, "Our results demonstrate the potential value of examining long-term meat consumption in assessing cancer risk and strengthen the evidence that prolonged high consumption of red and processed meat may increase the risk of cancer in the distal portion of the large intestine."

Studies from The Netherlands, and Iowa in the U.S. have focused on the association of heme iron with colon cancer. The Netherlands Cohort Study (Balder et al. 2006) concluded, "Our data suggested an elevated risk of colon cancer in men with increasing intake of heme iron and decreasing intake of chlorophyll."

Lee and coworkers reported results of the Iowa Women's Health Study (Lee et al. 2004a, 2004b, 2004c, 20005a, 2005b; Lee and Jacobs 2005). Lee et al. stated (2004a), "Our results suggest that intake of dietary heme iron is associated with an increased risk of proximal colon cancer, especially among women who drink (alcohol), but that dietary zinc intake is associated with a decreased risk of both proximal and distal colon cancer."

A study from France implicated high dietary iron and copper in colorectal cancer (Senesse et al. 2004). Nelson (2001) reviewed the association of iron and colorectal cancer risk, concluding, "Because iron is broadly supplemented in the American diet, the benefits of iron supplementation need to be measured against the long-term risks of increased iron exposure, one of which may be increased risk of colorectal cancer." Cross and Sinha (2004) suggested that "red meat may be associated with colorectal cancer by contributing to N-nitroso compound exposure.... Meats cooked at high temperatures contain other potential mutagens in the form of heterocyclic amines and polycyclic aromatic hydrocarbons." As previously discussed, iron is necessary for activating heterocyclic amines and polycyclic aromatic hydrocarbons to form their carcinogenic derivatives.

Experimental Studies

> *"A diet high in fat and iron is known as a risk factor for cancer epidemiology."*   (Sawa et al. 1998.)

Due to overwhelming epidemiological evidence that eating red meat and processed meat is associated with colorectal cancer, many experimental studies have attempted to determine the role of iron in colorectal carcinogenesis. All of these studies implicate redox cycling of iron in colon carcinogenesis. Some of these will now be reviewed in chronological order.

Nelson et al. (1989) examined the effect of parenteral and oral iron in a series of studies on rats in which dimethylhydrazine was used to initiate colorectal carcinogenesis. Both parenteral and oral iron augmented tumor incidence. Phytic acid, which binds iron, was found to reverse the augmenting effect of oral iron on tumor incidence. The studies indicated that iron's effect on colorectal tumor induction takes place during the promotional phase of carcinogenesis and not during initiation.

Babbs (1990) reviewed evidence that suggested that intracolonic production of oxygen radicals play a role in colon carcinogenesis, and concluded, "Intracolonic free radical formation may explain the high incidence of cancer in the colon and rectum, compared to other regions of the GI tract, as well as the observed correlations of a higher incidence of colon cancer with red meat in the diet, which increases stool iron, and with excessive fat in the diet, which may increase the fecal content of procarcinogens and bile pigments."

Kuratko (1998) reported a decrease of manganese superoxide dismutase activity in rats fed high levels of iron during colon carcinogenesis. Manganese superoxide dismutase aids in the removal of the superoxide ion generated by redox cycling of iron. The study suggested that reduced manganese superoxide dismutase induced by dietary iron may be one mechanism that allows carcinogenic foreign chemicals (xenobiotics) to induce colon cancer risk.

Sawa et al. (1998) examined the possible implications of lipid peroxyl radicals generated from fatty acids and heme-iron in DNA damage with subsequent colon cancer. In this animal model, simultaneous feeding of a fat diet and heme-iron produced a significant increase in the incidence of colon cancer compared with a diet without hemoglobin.

Sesink et al. (1999) discovered the presence of a cytotoxic substance in the fecal water from heme-fed rats. This suggested to the authors that "in heme-fed rats colonic mucosa is damaged by the intestinal contents. This results in compensatory hyperproliferation of the epithelium, which increases the risk for colon cancer."

Lund et al. (2001) studied lipid peroxidation in the intestinal mucosa in rats with chronic iron exposure. Their experiment demonstrated that chronic exposure to high levels of iron fortification increases oxidative damage in the rat large intestine.

Valko et al. (2001) examined the hypothesis that bile acids, vitamins K, iron, and oxygen interact to induce an oncogenic effect in the colon by generation of free radicals. They developed a model in which reduced K vitamins initiate superoxide radical generation leading to iron redox cycling in stem colon cells.

Stone et al. (2002) studied the influence of dietary iron on oxidative stress in the colon, and reported that high levels of dietary iron were found to promote oxidative stress in the feces and colonocytes.

Pierre et al. (2006) identified a marker for colon cancer risk associated with heme intake. The marker is a chemical known as 1,4-dihydroxynonane mercapturic acid.

Cancer Cells Require More Iron than Normal Cells

The contemporary concept of carcinogenesis is that cancer development proceeds in three stages: 1) initiation; 2) promotion; and 3) progression. The initiation phase involves mutagenic changes in DNA. The promotion phase involves transformation of mutated cells and their aggregation. Promotion is a relatively long process and usually continues for many years after initiation. Once the initiated and promoted cells begin to aggregate, the invasive progression phase begins and mutated cells continue to reproduce more and more rapidly. Iron is involved in cancer initiation and promotion by way of oxygen radical generation.

However, the role of iron in cancer progression is quite different. Because the progression phase is accompanied by rapid reproduction of cancerous cells to form the growing tumor mass, cancer cells require more iron than do normal cells. Recall that transferrin carries iron(III) in blood serum and delivers the iron to cells by attaching to receptors on the surface of the cell. The cell internalizes transferrin, the iron is released, and the transferrin is returned to the serum. Cancer cells have many more transferrin receptors than do normal cells and are more capable of trapping transferrin and scavenging its iron. In this way, the cancer cell creates a layer of cells surrounding the tumor that are "anemic"—they don't have enough iron to function well. This allows the rapidly-dividing, iron-satisfied cancer cells to become more invasive and to destroy the iron-deficient anemic cells that surround it.

Transferrin Receptors

Increased numbers of transferrin receptors have been reported on human mammary carcinomas (Vandewalle et al. 1985; Kosano and Takatani 1990; Reizenstein 1991; Shterman et al. 1991; Elliott et al. 1993; Inoue et al. 1993); prostate cancer (Keer et al. 1990); bladder cancer (Başar et al. 1991) and colon cancer (Drewinko et al. 1987).

Başar et al. (1991) reported studies on transferrin receptors in bladder cancer and reported, "Patients with low grade superficial tumours showing transferrin activity had a higher recurrence rate than those with no transferrin activity. It was concluded that transferrin activity in low grade superficial bladder tumours is a useful marker for predicting the recurrence rate."

In a unique study of drug-resistant and drug-sensitive cancer cells, Barabas and Faulk (1993) reported that drug-resistant cells have more transferrin receptors than drug-sensitive cells.

Applications of Increased Transferrin Receptors

Since the turn of this century, there has been a good deal of interest in using the increased numbers of transferrin receptors on cancer cells as a chemotherapeutic approach to cancer. The concept is to attach cancer-killing drugs to transferrin and introduce the transferrin-cancer-killing drug complex to the cancer cells. This branch of cancer chemotherapy is so new that its applications are only beginning to be explored.

Artemisinin is an important drug with anti-cancer properties; however, some cancer cells are resistant to artemisinin. Nonetheless, when artemisinin is attached to transferrin, drug resistance can be overcome. Several laboratories have experimented in developing a transferrin-bound artemisinin for cancer treatment (Sadava et al. 2002; Lai et al. 2005a and 2005b; Nakase et al. 2007). Targeted delivery of other cancer-killing drugs by attaching the drug to transferrin is under investigation. Adriamycin has been incorporated into transferrin liposomes (Lopez-Barcons et al. 2005). Transferrin-conjugated paclitaxel-loaded nanoparticles have also been used (Sahoo and Labhasetwar 2005).

Yang et al. (2001) used a drug that targets the gene that makes the transferrin receptor. The drug slows down production of transferrin receptors, making the cancer cells more susceptible to other cancer-killing drugs. Pun et al. (2004) extended this work by developing transferrin-modified nanoparticles containing an enzyme that destroys the cancer cell's ability to make transferrin receptors.

Lactoferrin

Lactoferrin is found in secretions of lachrymal glands and mammary glands and in secretions of respiratory, gastrointestinal, and genital tracts. Lactoferrin acts in conjunction with lysozyme as a primary defense against invading organisms. Lysozyme cuts holes in the membranes of microbes, and lactoferrin binds iron so that surviving microbes cannot survive. The relationship between lactoferrin and infection has been known for many years.

The anti-cancer properties of lactoferrin have been discovered more recently. Since 2000, numerous studies have demonstrated lactoferrin's anti-cancer properties (Tauda and Sekine 2000; Tsuda et al. 2000, 2002; Shimamura et al. 2004; Varadhachary et al. 2004; Mader et al. 2006; Wolf et al. 2007; Kanwar et al. 2008). Chandra and Mohan and their various collaborators have studied the combined effect of lactoferrin and black tea polyphenols in prevention of hamster buccal pouch carcinogenesis (Chandra et al. 2006a, 2006b; Mohan et al. 2007, 2008). Anti-papillomavirus properties of lactoferrin have been recently discovered (Drobni et al. 2004; Mistry et al. 2007). Artym et al. (2003) reported that orally administered lactoferrin can restore humoral response in immunocompromised mice.

Cancer-Associated Anemia

The vast majority of cancer victims will develop anemia, in part, due to the cancer cell's voracious appetite for iron, and, in part due to iron withholding as a defense against disease. For reviews of the anemia of chronic disease, refer to: Bullen and Griffiths (1987); Griffiths and Bullen (1987); Weiss et al. (2005); Ward et al. (2005); Weinberg (1996, 2002, 2005, 2007); Yamauchi et al. (2006). Volumes have been written on this subject, some of which will be discussed later.

For now, here is a brief overview of the way the iron homeostasis responds to cancer cells. Hepcidin is the iron-regulatory protein that is made in the liver and causes a decrease in iron absorption and induces iron sequestration in the reticuloendothelial macrophages. A substance known as p53, a tumor-suppressor that regulates genes involved in growth arrest, cell death (apoptosis), and DNA repair, is secreted by normal cells. P53 increases synthesis of hepcidin, thereby causing a decrease in iron absorption accompanied by sequestration of iron into ferritin where it cannot be used by the cancer cells.

Cancer cells cause a perturbation of the p53 pathway, and this is a hallmark of most human cancer cells. It therefore has been suggested that hepcidin induction by p53 is one of the mechanisms involved in the anemia accompanying cancer (Weizer-Stern et al. 2007).

Conclusions

Iron is a primary carcinogen: Dietary iron overload causes hepatocellular carcinoma in humans and laboratory animals.

Iron is a co-carcinogen: Iron activates many xenobiotics, resulting in carcinogenicity.

Iron is a synergistic carcinogen: Iron has a multiplicative carcinogenic effect in conjunction with alcohol, aflatoxin, hepatitis B, hepatitis C, HIV, and papillomavirus.

Iron is a cumulative carcinogen: Iron accumulates with age; once excess iron is absorbed, the human body has no physiological mechanism for removing it.

Iron is a complete carcinogen: Iron is involved in all three phases of cancer development: initiation, promotion, and progression.

REFERENCES

Abalea V, Cillard J, Dubos MP, Anger JP, Cillard P, Morel I. 1998. Iron-induced oxidative DNA damage and its repair in primary rat hepatocyte culture. Carcinogenesis. 19(6):1053-9.

Alexander J, Tung BY, Croghan A, Kowdley KV. 2007. Effect of iron depletion on serum markers of fibrogenesis, oxidative stress and serum liver enzymes in chronic hepatitis C: results of a pilot study. Liver Int. 27(2):268-73.

Antoine D, Braun P, Cervoni P, Schwartz P, Lamy P. 1979. Le cancer bronique des mineurs de fer de Lorraine peut-il étre consideré comme un maladie professionelle? Rev Fr Mal Respir. 7:63-5.

Artym J, Zimecki M, Paprocka M, Kruzel ML. 2003. Orally administered lactoferrin restores humoral immune response in immunocompromised mice. Immunol Lett. 89(1):9-15.

Asare GA, Bronz M, Naidoo V, Kew MC. 2007. Interactions between aflatoxin B1 and dietary iron overload in hepatic mutagenesis. Toxicology.

234(3):157-66.

Asare GA, Mossanda KS, Kew MC, Peterson AC, Kahler-Venter CP, Siziba K. 2006a. Hepatocellular carcinoma caused by iron overload: a possible mechanism of direct hepatocarcinogenicity. Toxicology 219(1-3):41-52.

Asare GA, Paterson AC, Kew MC, Khan S, Mossanda KS. 2006b. Iron-free neoplastic nodules and hepatocellular carcinoma without cirrhosis in Wistar rats fed a diet high in iron. J Pathol. 208(1):82-90.

Aust A, Lund L, Chao C, Park S, Fang R. 2000. Role of iron in cellular effects of asbestos. Inhalation Toxicol. 12:S75S-80S.

Avunduk AM, Yardimci S, Avunduk MC, Kurnaz, L, Cengiz M. 2000. A possible mechanism of X-ray-induced injury to the lens. Jpn J Ophthalmol. 44(1):88-91.

Babbs CF. 1990. Free radicals and the etiology of colon cancer. Free Radic Biol Med. 8(2):191-200.

Bacon BR, Britton RS. 1989. Hepatic injury in chronic iron overload. Role of lipid peroxidation. Chem Biol Interact. 70(3-4):183-226.

Bacon BR, O'Neill R, Britton RS. 1993. Hepatic mitochondrial energy production in rats with chronic iron overload. Gastroenterology. 105(4):1134-40.

Bacon BR. 1997. Iron and hepatitis C. Gut. 41:127-8.

Baird WH, Hooven LA, Mahadevan B. 2005. Carcinogenic polycyclic aromatic hydrocarbon-DNA adducts and mechanism of action. Environ Mol Mutagen. 45(2-3):106-14.

Balder HF, de Vogel J, Jansen MCJf, Weijenberg MP, van den Brandt, PA, Westenbrink S, van der Meer R, Goldbohm RA. 2006. Heme and chlorophyll intake and risk of colorectal cancer in the Netherlands cohort study. Cancer Epidemiol Biomarkers Prev. 15(4):717-25.

Baldys A, Aust AE. 2005. Role of iron in inactivation of epidermal growth factor receptor after asbestos treatment of human lung and pleural target cells. Am J Resp Cell Molecular Biol. (32):436-42.

Ball BR, Smith KR, Vernath JM, Aust AE. 2000. Bioavailability of iron from coal fly ash: mechanisms of mobilization and of biological effects. Inhal Toxicol. 12(Suppl 4):209-25.

Barton AL, Banner BR, Cable EE, Bonkovsky HL. 1995. Distribution of iron in the liver predicts the response of chronic hepatitis C infection to interferon therapy. Am J Clin Pathol. 103:419-24.

Başar I, Ayhan A, Bircan K, Ergen A, Taşar C. 1991. Transferrin receptor activity as a marker in transitional cell carcinoma of the bladder. Br J

Urol. 67(2):165-8.

Benhar M, Engelberg D, Levitzki A. 2002. ROS, stress-activated kinases and stress signaling in cancer. EMBO Rep. 3:420-25.

Benz CC, Clarke CA, Moore II, DH. 2003. Geographic excess of estrogen receptor-positive breast cancer. Cancer Epidem, Biomarkers and Prevention. 12:1525-7.

Bissett D, Chaterjee R, Hannon DP. 1991. Chronic ultraviolet radiation-increase in skin iron and the photoprotective effect of topically applied iron chelators. Photochem Photobiol. 54:215-13.

Bissett DL, McBride JF. 1996. Synergistic topical photoprotection by a combination of the iron chelator 2-furlicioxime and sunscreen. Am Acad Dermatol. 35(4):546-9.

Bonkovsky HL, Lambrecht RW, Shan Y. 2003. Iron as a co-morbid factor in nonhemochromatotic liver disease. Alcohol 30(2):137-44.

Bonkovsky HL, Lambrecht RW. 2000. Iron-induced liver injury. Clin Liver Dis. 4(vi-vii):409-29.

Bonkovsky HL. 1991. Iron and the liver. Am J Med Sci. 301:32-43.

Boyd JT, Doll R, Faulds JS, Leiper J. 1970. Cancer of the lung in iron ore (hematite) miners. Br J Indust Med. 27:97-105.

Brittenham GM. 2003. Iron chelators and iron toxicity. Alcohol. 30(2):151-8.

Britton RS, Bacon BR, Recknagel RO. 1987. Lipid peroxidation and associated hepatic organelle dysfunction in iron overload. 45(2-4):207-39.

Britton RS, Bacon BR. 1994. Role of free radicals in liver disease and hepatic fibrosis. Hepatogastroenterology. 41(4):343-8.

Britton RS, Ramm GA, Olynyk J, Singh R, O'Neill R, Bacon BR. 1994. Pathophysiology of iron toxicity. Adv Exp Med Biol. 356:239-53.

Britton RS. 1996. Metal-induced hepatotoxicity. Semin Liver Dis. 16(1):3-12.

Bullen JJ, Griffiths E, eds. 1987. *Iron and Infection.* John Wiley and Sons, Chichester, New York, Brisbane, Toronto, Singapore.

Campbell JA. 1940. Effects of precipitated silica and of iron oxide on the incidence of primary lung tumors in mice. Br Med J. 2:275-80.

Carter RL, Mitchley BC, Roe FJ. 1968. Induction of tumors in mice and rats with ferric sodium gluconate and iron dextran glycerol glycoside. Br J Cancer. 22(3):521-26.

Carter RL. 1969. Early development of injection-site sarcomas in rats: a study of tumours induced by iron-dextran. Br J Cancer. 23(3):559-66.

Case BW, Ip MP, Padilla M, Kleinerman J. 1986. Asbestos effects on superoxide production. An in vitro study of hamster alveolar macrophages. Environ Res. 39(2):299-306.

Cavalieri EL, Rogan EG, Li K, Todorovic R, Ariese F, Jankowiak R, Gruber N, Small GJ. 2005. Identification and quantification of depurinating DNA adducts formed in mouse skin treated with dibenzo[*a,l*]pyrine (DB[*a,l*]P) or its metabolites and in rat mammary gland treated with DB[*a,l*]P. Chem Res Toxicol. 18:976-83.

Cederbaum AI. 1992. Iron and ethanol-induced tissue damage: Generation of reactive oxygen intermediates and possible mechanisms for their role of alcohol liver toxicity. In: *Iron and Human Disease.* Lauffer RB, ed. Boca Raton, Ann Arbor, London, Tokyo: CRC Press, pp 419-46.

———— 2003. Iron and CYP2E1-dependent oxidative stress and toxicity. Alcohol. 30(2):115-20.

Chandra Mohan KB, Devraj H, Prathiba D, Hara Y, Nagini S. 2006. Antiproliferative apoptosis inducing effect of lactoferrin and black tea polyphenol combination on hamster buccal pouch carcinogenesis. Biochim Biophys Acta. 1760(10):1536-44.

Chandra Mohan KB, Kumaraguruparan R, Prathiba D, Nagini S. 2006. Modulation of xenobiotic-metabolizing enzymes and redox status during chemoprevention of hamster buccal carcinogenesis by bovine lactoferrin. Nutrition. 22(9):940-6.

Chandra RK. 1965. The risk of sarcomatous change after iron-dextran therapy. Indian J Pediatr. 32:75-7.

Chao A, Thun MJ, Connell CJ, McCullough ML, Jacobs EJ, Flanders WD, Rodriguez C, Sinha R, Calle EE. 2005. Meat consumption and risk of colorectal cancer. JAMA. 293(2):233-4.

Chao CC, Lund LG, Zinn KR, Aust AE. 1994. Iron mobilization from crocidolite asbestos by human lung carcinoma cells. Arch Biochem Biophys. 314(2):384-91.

Chao CC, Park SH, Aust AE. 1996. Participation of nitric oxide and iron in the oxidation of DNA in asbestos-treated human lung epithelial cells. Arch Biochem Biophys. 326(1):152-7.

Churg A, Hobson J, Berean K, Wright J. 1989. Scavengers of active oxygen species prevent cigarette smoke-induced asbestos fiber penetration in rat tracheal explants. Am J Pathol. 135(4):599-603.

Conway K, Parrish E, Edmiston SN, Tolbert D, Tse C-K, Moorman P, Newman B, Millikan RC. 2007. Risk factors for breast cancer characterized by the estrogen receptor alpha A908G (K303R) mutation. Breast

Cancer Research. 9:R36 (Available online at *http://breast-cancer-research. com/content/9/3/R36*).

Cross AJ, Gunter MJ, Wood RJ, Pietinen P, Taylor PR, Virtamo J, Albanes D, Sinha R. 2006. Iron and colorectal cancer risk in the alpha-tocopherol, beta-carotene cancer prevention study. Int J Cancer. 118(12):147-52.

Cross AJ, Sinha R. 2004. Meat-related mutagens/carcinogens in the etiology of colorectal cancer. Environ Mol Mutagen. 44(1):44-55.

Crowley JD, Still WJ. 1960. Metastatic carcinoma at the site of injection of iron-dextran complex. Br Med J. 1(5183):1411-12.

Cui Y, Vogt S, Olson N, Glass AG, Rohan TE. 2007. Levels of zinc, selenium, calcium, and iron in benign breast tissue and risk of subsequent breast cancer. 16(8):2173.

Cyrus-David MS, Strom SS. 2001. Chemoprevention of breast cancer with selective estrogen receptor modulators: views from broadly diverse focus groups of women with elevated risk for breast cancer. Psychooncology. 10(6):521-33.

Dai K. Koam K. Bpsland M, Frenkel K, Bernhardt G, Huang X. 2007. Roles of hormone replacement therapy and iron in proliferation of breast epithelial cells with different estrogen and progesterone receptor status. Breast. Oct. 8; [Epub ahead of print].

De Feo TM, Fargion S, Duca L, Cesana BM, Boncinelli L, Lozza P, Cappellini MD, Fiorelli G. 2001. Non-transferrin-bound iron in alcohol abusers. Alcohol Clin Exp Res. 25(10):1494-9.

Deugnier Y, Turlin B. 2001. Iron and hepatocellular carcinoma. J Gastroenterol Hepatol. 16(5):491-4.

——— 2002. Iron overload disorders. Clin Liv Dis. 6(2):481-96.

——— 2007. Pathology of hepatic iron overload. World J Gastroenterol. 13(35):4755-4760.

Deugnier Y. 2003. Iron and liver cancer. Alcohol. 30(2):145-50.

Dey A, Cederbaum AL. 2006. Alcohol and oxidative liver injury. Hepatology. 43:S63-S74.

Distante S, Bjoro K, Hellum KB, Myrvang B, Berg JP, Skaug K, Raknerud N, Bell H. 2002. Raised serum ferritin predicts non-response to interferon and ribavirin treatment in patients with chronic hepatitis C infection. Liver 22(3):269-75.

Donaldson K, Cullen RT. 1984. Chemiluminescence of asbestos-activated macrophages. Br J Exp Pathol. 65(1):81-90.

Donaldson K, Slight J, Hannant D, Bolton RE. 1985. Increased release of hydrogen peroxide and superoxide anion from asbestos-primed macrophages. Effect of hydrogen peroxide on the functional activity of alpha 1-protease inhibitor. Inflammation. 9(2):139-47.

Drewinko B, Moskwa P, Reuben J. 1987. Expression of transferrin receptors is unrelated to proliferative status in cultured human colon cancer cells. Anticancer Res. 7(2):139-41.

Dreyfus J. 1936. Lung carcinoma among siblings who have inhaled dust containing iron oxides during their youth. Clin Med. 30:256-60.

Drobni P, Näslund J, Evander M. 2004. Lactoferrin inhibits human papilomavirus binding and uptke in vitro. Antiviral Res. 64(1):63-8.

Dunkel VC, San RH, Seifried HE, Whittaker P. 1999. Genotoxicity of iron compounds in Salmonella typhimurium and L5178Y mouse lymphoma cells. Environ Mol Mutagen. 33(1):28-41.

Dunne JR, Gannon CJ, Osborn TM, Taylor MD, Maione DL, Napolitano LM. 2002. Preoperative anemia in colon cancer: assessment of risk factors. Am Surg. 68(6):582-7.

Edling C. 1982. Lung cancer and smoking in a group of iron ore miners. Am J Indust Med. 3:191-99.

Eichbaum Q, Foran S, Dziks S. 2003. Is iron gluconate really safer than iron dextran? Blood. 101(9):3756-7.

Elliott RL, Elliott MC, Wang F, Head JF. 1993. Breast carcinoma and the role of iron metabolism. A cytochemical, tissue culture, and ultrastructural study. Ann NY Acad Sci. 698:159-66.

Elstner EF. Schütz W, Vogl G. 1986. Enhancement of enzyme-catalyzed production of reactive oxygen species by suspensions of "crocidolite" asbestos fibres. Free Radic Res Commun. 1(6):355-9.

———— 1988. Cooperative stimulation by sulfite and crocidolite asbestos fibers on enzyme catalyzed production of reactive oxygen species. Arch Toxicol. 62(6):424-7.

English DR, MacInnis RJ, Hodge AM, Hopper JL, Haydon AM, Giles GG. 2004. Red meat, chicken, and fish consumption and risk of colorectal cancer. Cancer Epidemiol Biomarkers Prev. 2004. 13(9):1509-14.

Fang R, Aust AE. 1997. Induction of ferritin synthesis in human lung epithelial cells treated with crocidolite asbestos. Arch Biochem Biophys. 340(2):369-75.

Fargion S, Fracanzani AL, Sampietro M, Molteni V, Boldorini R, Mattioli M, Cesana B, Lunghi G, Piperno A, Valsecchi C, Fiorelli G. 1997. Liver iron influences the response to interferon alpha therapy in chronic hepatitis C. Eur J Gastroenterol Hepatol. 9(5):497-503.

Feelders RA, Vreugdenhil G, Eggermont AM, Kuiper-Kramer PA, van Ejk HG, Swaak AJ. 1998. Regulation of iron metabolism in the acute-phase response: interferon gamma and tumour necrosis factor alpha induce hypoferraemia, ferritin production and a decrease in circulating transferrin receptors in cancer patients. Eur J Clin Invest. 28(7):520-7.

Ferrali M, Signorini C, Sugherini L, Pompella A, Lodovici M, Caciotti B, Camporti M. 1997. Release of free, redox-active iron in the liver and DNA oxidative damage following phenylhydrazine intoxication. Biochem Pharmacol. 53(11):1743-51.

Fletcher LM, Bridle KR, Crawford DH. 2003. Effect of alcohol on iron storage diseases of the liver. Best Pract Res Clin Gastroenterol. 17(4):663-77.

Fletcher LM, Powell LW. 2003. Hemochromatosis and alcoholic liver disease. Alcohol. 30(2):131-6.

Food and Nutrition Board. 1993. *Iron Deficiency Anemia: Recommended Guidelines for the Prevention, Detection, and Management Among U.S. Children and Women of Childbearing Age.* Earl R, Woteki CE, eds. Washington: National Academy Press.

———— 2001. *Dietary Reference Intakes for Vitamin A, Vitamin K, Arsenic, Boron, Chromium, Copper, Iodine, Iron, Manganese, Molybdenum, Nickel, Silicon, Vanadium, and Zinc.* Washington: National Academy Press.

Fujita N, Horiike S, Sugimoto R, Tanaka H, Iwasa M, Kobayashi Y, Hasegawa K, Ma N, Kawanishi S, Adachi Y, Kaito M. 2007a. Hepatic oxidative DNA damage correlates with iron overload in chronic hepatitis C patients. 42(3):353-62.

Fujita N, Sugimoto R, Urawa N, Araki J, Mifuji R, Yamamoto M, Horiike S, Tanaka H, Iwasa M, Kobayashi Y, Adachi Y, Kaito M. 2007b. Hepatic iron accumulation is associated with disease progression and resistance to interferon/ribavirin combination therapy in chronic hepatitis C. J Gastroenterol Hepatol. 22(11):1886-93.

Furst A. 1960. Metals in tumors. In: *Metal Binding in Medicine.* Steven MJ, Johnson LA, eds. Philadelphia: JB Lippincott, p 346.

Furutani T, Hino K, Okuda M, Gondo T, Nishina S, Kitase A, Korenaga M, Xiao SY, Weinman SA, Lemon SM, Sakaida I, Okita K. 2006. Hepatic iron overload induces hepatocellular carcinoma in transgenic mice expressing the hepatitis C virus polyprotein. Gastroenterology. 130(7):2087-98.

Gackowski D, Kruszewski M, Banaszkiewicz Z, Jawien A, Olinski R. 2002. Lymphocyte labile iron pool, plasma iron, transferrin saturation and ferritin levels in colon cancer parients. Acta Biochimica Polonica. 49 1:269-72.

Galey JB, Destrée O, Dumats J, Gébard S, Tachon P. 2000. Protection against oxidative damage by iron chelators: effect of lipophilic analogues and prodrugs of N,N-bis(3,4,5-trimethoxylbenzyl) ethylene-diamine N,N-diacetic acid (OR10141). J Med Chem. 43:1418-21.

Garcon G, Gosset P, Maunit B, Zerimech F, Creusy C, Muller JF, Shirall P. 2004a. Influence of iron ($^{56}Fe_2O_3$ or $^{54}Fe_2O_3$) in the upregulation of chtochrome P4501A1 by benzo[a]pyrene in the respiratory tract of Sprague-Dawley rats. App. Toxicol. 24(3):249-56.

Garcon G, Gosset P, Zerimech F, Grave-Descampiaux B, Shirali P. 2004b. effect of Fe_2O_3on the capacity of benzo[a]pyrene to induce polycyclic aromatic hydrocarbon-metabolizind enzymes in the respiratory tract of Sprague-Dawley rats. Toxicol Lett. 150(2):179-89.

Giler S, Moroz C. 1978. The significance of ferritin in malignant diseases. Biomedicine. 28(4):203-6.

Gillie A. 1964. Iron-dextran and sarcomata. Br Med J. 1(5398):1593-4.

Giuffrida G, Condorelli M, Filocamo G Jr, Migliau G, Pugliese F, Basile U. 1964. Carcinogenic risk of iron-dextran. Br Med J. 1(5398):1583-4.

Gloyne SR. 1935. Two cases of squamous carcinoma of the lung occurring in asbestosis. Tubercle. 17:5-10.

Goodglick LA, Kane AB. 1986. Role of reactive oxygen metabolites in crocidolite asbestos toxicity to mouse macrophages. Cancer Res. 46(11):5558-66.

———— 1990. Cytotoxicity of long and short crocidolite asbestos fibers in vitro and in vivo. Cancer Res. 50(16):5153-63.

Griffiths E, Bullen JJ. 1987. Iron-binding proteins and host defence. In: *Iron and Infection.* Chichester, New York, Brisbane, Toronto, Singapore: John Wiley and Sons, p 171-211.

Grotto HZ. 2008. Anaemia of cancer: an overview of mechanisms involved in its pathogenesis. Med Oncol. 25(1):12-21.

Gunel-Ozcan A, Alyilmaz-Bekmez , Guler EN, Guc D. 2006. HFE H63D mutation frequency shows an increae in Turkish women with breast cancer. BMC Cancer. 6:37.

Guo WD, Chow WH, Zheng W, Li JY, Blot WJ. 1994. Diet, serum markers and breast cancer mortality in Chiona. Jpn J Cancer Res. 85(6):572-7.

Haddow A, Horning ES. 1960. On the carcinogenicity of an iron-dextran complex. J Natl Cancer Inst. 24:109-47.

Haddow A, Roe FJ, Mitchley BC. 1964. Induction of sarcomata in rabbits by intramuscular injection of iron-dextran ("Imferon"). Br Med J. 1(5398):1593-4.

Halliwell B, Zhao K, Whiteman M. 2000. The gastrointestinal tract: a major site of antioxidant action? Free Radic Res. 33(6):819-30.

Hansen K, Mossman BT. 1987. Generation of superoxide (O_2^-) from alveolar macrophages exposed to asbestiform and nonfibrous particles. Cancer Res. 47(6):1681-6.

Hardy JA, Aust AE. 1995. The effect of iron binding on the ability of crocidolite asbestos to catalyze DNA single-strand breaks. Carcinogenesis. 16(2):319-25.

Harrison-Findik DD, Klein E, Crist C, Evans J, Timchenko N, Gollan J. 2007. Iron-mediated regulation of liver hepcidin expression in rats and mice is abolished by alcohol. Hepatology. 46(6):1979-85.

Harrison-Findik DD, Schafer D, Klein E, Timchenko NA, Kulaksiz H, Clemens D, Fein E, Andropoulos B, Pantopoulos K, Gollan J. 2006. Alcohol metabolism-mediated oxidative stress down-regulates hepcidin transcription and leads to increased duodenal iron transporter expression. J Biol Chem. 281(32):22974-82.

Harrison-Findik DD. 2007. Role of alcohol in the regulation of iron metabolism. World J Gastroenterol. 13(37):4925-30.

Hileti D, Panayiotidis P, Hoffbrand AV. 1995. Iron chelators induce apoptosis in proliferating cells. Br J Haematol. 89:181-7.

Hong CC, Ambrosone CB, Ahn J, Choi JY, McCullough ML, Stevens VL, Rodriguez C, Thun MJ, Calle EE. 2007. Genetic variability in iron-related oxidative stress pathways (Nrf2, NQ01, NOS3. and OH-1), iron intake and risk of postmenopausal breast cancer. Cancer Epidemiol Bio-markers Prev. 16(9):1784-94.

Huang X. 2003. Iron overload and its association with cancer risk in humans: evidence for iron as a carcinogenic metal. Mutat Res. 533:153-71.

IARC. 1973. *Some Inorganic and Organomatellic Compounds*. IARC Monographs of the Evaluation of Carcinogenic Risk to Humans. Vol. 2. Lyon France: International Agency for Research on Cancer. p 181.

Icso J, Szollosova M, Sorahan T. 1994. Lung cancer among iron ore miners in east Slovakia: a case-control study. Occup Environ Med. 51:642-3.

Iguchi H, Kojo S. 1989. Possible generation of hydrogen peroxide and lipid peroxidation of erythrocyte membrane by asbestos: cytotoxic mechanism of asbestos. Biochem Int. 18(5):981-90.

Inoue T, Cavanaugh PG, Steck PA, Brünner N, Nicholson GL. 1993. Differences in transferrin response and numbers of transferrin receptors in rat and human mammary carcinoma lines of different metastatic potentials. J Cell Physiol. 156(1):212-7.

Ioannou GN, Weiss NS, Kowdley KV. 2007. Relationship between transferrin-iron saturation, alcohol consumption, and the incidence of cirrhosis and liver cancer. Clin Gastroenterol Hepatol. 5(5):624-9.

Jacobs A, Jones B, Ricketts C, Bulbrook RD, Wang DY. 1976. Serum ferritin concentration in early breast cancer. Br J Cancer. 34(3):286-90.

Kabat GC, Miller AB, Jain M, Rohan TE. 2007. Dietary iron and heme iron intake and risk of breast cancer: a prospective cohort study. Cancer Epidemiol Biomarkers Prev. 16(6):1306-8.

Kabat GC, Rohan TE. 2007. Does excess iron play a role in breast carcinogenesis? an unresolved hypothesis. Cancer Causes Control. 18(10):1047-53.

Kadota K, Wada T, Watatani M, Houjou T, Mori N, Yasutomi M. 1991. [The elevation of serum iron level with oral administration of medoprogesterone acetate (MPA) in patients with brease cancer.] Gan To Kagaku Ryoho. 18(6):983-7. [Article in Japanese]

Kallianpur AR, Hall LD, Yadav M, Christman BW, Dittus RS, Haines JL, Parl FR, Summar ML. 2004. Increased prevalence of the DFE C282Y hemochromatosis allele in women with breast cancer. Cancer Epidemiol Biomarkers Prev. 13:205-12.

Kallianpur AR, Lee SA, Gao YT, Lu W, Zheng Y, Ruan ZX, Dai Q, Gu K, Shu XO, Zheng W. 2008. Dietary animal-derived iron and fat intake and breast cancer risk in the Shanghai Breast Cancer Study. Breast Cancer Res Treat. 107(1):123-32.

Kallianpur AR, Lee SA, Gao YT, Lu W, Zheng ZX, Dai Q, Gu K, Shu XO, Zheng W. 2007. Dietary animal-derived iron and fat intake and breast cancer risk in the Shanghai Breast Cancer Study. Breast Cancer Res Treat. Mar 13. [Epub ahead of print]

Kamp DW, Graceffa P, Pryor WA, Weitzman SA. 1992. The role of free radicals in asbestos-induced diseases. 12(4):293-315.

Kamp DW, Israbian VA, Preusen SE, Zhang CX, Weitzman SA. 1995. Asbestos causes DNA strand breaks in cultured pulmonary epithelial cells: role of iron-catalysed free radicals. Am J Physiol. 268:L471-80.

Kang JO, Jones C, Brothwell B. 1998. Toxicity associated with iron overload found in hemochromatosis: possible mechanism in a rat model.

Clin Lab Sci. 11(6):350-4.

Kanwar JR, Palmano KP, Sun X, Kanwar RK, Gupta R, Haggarty N, Rowan A, Ram S, Krissansen GW. 'Ion-saturated' lactoferrin is a potent natural adjuvant for augmenting cancer chemotherapy. Immunol Cell Biol. [Epub ahead of print].

Kato I, Dnistrian AM, Schwartz M, Toniolo P, Koenig K, Shore RE, Zeleniuch-Jacquotte A, Akhmedkhanov A, Riboli E. 1999. Iron intake, body iron stores and colorectal cancer risk in women: a nested case-control study. Int J Cancer. 80(5):693-8.

Kato J, Miyanishi K, Kobune M, Nakamura T, Takada K, Takimoto R, Kawano Y, Takahashi S, Takahashi M, Sato Y, Takayama T, Niitsu Y. 2007. Long-term phlebotomy with low-iron diet therapy lowers risk of development of hepatocellular carcinoma from chronic hepatitis C. Gastroenterol. 42(10):830-6.

Keer HN, Koziowski JM, Lee C, McEwan RN, Grayhack JT. 1990. Elevated transferrin receptor content in human prostate cancer cell lines assessed in vitro and in vivo. J Urol. 143(2):381-5.

Kew MC, Asare GA. 2007. Dietary overload in the African and hepatocellular carcinoma. 27(6):735-43.

Kitazawa M, Ishitsuka Y, Kobayashi M, Nakano T, Iwasaki K, Sakamoto K Arakane K, Suzuki T, Klingman LH. 2005. Protective effects of an antioxidant derived from serine and vitamin B6 on skin photoaging in hairless mice. Photochem Photobiol. 81:970-4.

Koerten HD, Brederoo P, Ginsel LA, Daems WT. 1986. The endocytosis of asbestos by mouse peritoneal macrophages and its long-term effect on iron accumulation and labyrinth formation. Eur J Cell Biol. 40(1):25-36.

Koerten HD, Hazekamp J, Kroon M, Daems WT. 1990. Asbestos body formation and iron accumulation in mouse peritoneal granulomas after the introduction of crocidolite asbestos fibers. Am J Pathol. 136(1):141-57.

Kokocińska D, Widala E, Donocik J, Nolewajka E. 1999. [The value of evalualting tumor markers: CA 15-3 and ferritin in blood serum of patients group as "high risk" for breast cancer.] Przegl Lek. 56(10):664-7. [Article in Polish]

Kong S, Davison AJ. 1981. The relative effectiveness of $\cdot OH$, H_2O_2, O_2^-, and reducing free radicals in causing damage to biomembranes. A study of radiation damage to erythrocyte ghosts using selective free radical scavengers. Biochem Biophys Acta. 640(1):313-25.

Kong S, Davison AJ, Bland J. 1981. Actions of gamma-radiation on resealed erythrocyte ghosts. A Comparison with intact erythrocytes and a study of the effects of oxygen. Int J Radiat Biol Relat Study Phys Chem Med. 40(1):19-29.

Kosano H, Takatani O. 1990. Increase of transferrin binding induced by an alkyl-lysophospholipid in breast cancer cells. J Lipid Mediat. 2(2):117-21.

Kucharzewski M, Braziewica J, Majewska U, Gózdz S. 2003. Iron concentrations in intestinal cancer tissue and in colon and rectum polyps. Biol Trace Elem Res. 95(1):19-28.

Kunz J. 1964. [Autoradiographic studies on mast cells in iron dextran-induced sarcoma.] Acta Biol Med Ger. 13:233-8. (German)

Kuratko CN. 1998. decrease of manganese superoxide dismutase activity in rats fed high levels of iron during colon carcinogenesis. Food Chem Toxicol. 36(9-10)819-24.

Kvam E, Hejmadi V, Ryter S, Pourzand C, Tyrrell RM. 2000. Heme oxygenase activity causes transient hypersensitivity to oxidative ultraviolet A radiation that depends on release of iron from heme. Free Radic Biol Med. 28(8):1191-6.

Lai H, Sasaki T, Singh NP. 2005a. Targeted treatment of cancer with artemisinin-tagged iron-carrying compounds. Expert Opin Ther Targets. 9(5):995-1007.9.

Lai H, Sasaki T, Singh NP, Messay A. 2005b. Effects of artemisinin-tagged holotransferin on cancer cells. Life Sci. 76(11):1267-79.

Larsson SC, Adami HO, Giovannucci E, Wolk A. 2005a. Correspondence. Re: Heme iron, zinc, alcohol consumption, and risk of colon cancer. J Natl Cancer Inst. 97(3):222-233.

Larsson SC, Rafter J, Holmberg L, Bergkvist L, Wolk A. 2004. Red meat consumption and risk of cancers of the proximal colon, distal colon and rectum: The Swedish Mammography Cohort. Int J Cancer. 113(5):829-34.

———— 2005b. Red meat consumption and risk of cancers of the proximal colon, distal colon and rectum: The Swedish Mammography Cohort. Int J Cancer. 113:829-34.

Lee DH, Anderson KE, Folsom AR, Jacobs DR Jr. 2005a. Heme iron, zinc and upper digestive tract cancer: the Iowa Women's Health Study. Int J Cancer. 117(4):643-7.

Lee DH, Anderson KE, Harnack LJ, Folsom AR, Jacobs DR Jr. 2004a. Heme iron, zinc, alcohol consumption, and colon cancer: Iowa Women's Health Study. J Natl Cancer Inst. 96:403-7.

Lee DH, Anderson KE, Harnack Lj, Folsom AR, Jacobs DR Jr. 2004b. Heme iron, zinc, alcohol consumption, and colon cancer: Iowa Women's Health Study. J Natl Cancer Inst. 96(5):403-7.

Lee DH, Jacobs DR Jr, Anderson KE. 2005b. Correspondence. Response Re: Heme iron, zinc, alcohol consumption, and risk of colon cancer. J Natl Cancer Inst. 97(3):233.

Lee DH, Jacobs DR Jr. 2005. Interaction among heme iron, zinc, and supplemental vitamin C intake on the risk of lung cancer: Iowa Women's Health Study. Nutr Cancer. 52(2):130-7.

Lee DH, Jacobs Jr DR, Folsom AR. 2004c. A hypothesis: interaction between supplemental iron intake and fermentation affecting the risk of colon cancer. The Iowa Women's Health Study. 48(1):1-5.

Li Z, Xia W, Fang B, Yan DH. 2001. Targeting HER-2/neu-overexpressing breast cancer cells by an antisense iron responsive element-directed gene expression. Cancer Let. 174(2):151-8.

Liehr JC, Jones JS. 2001. Role of iron in estrogen-induced cancer. Curr Med Chem. 8(7):839-49.

Lopez-Barcons LA, Polo D, Liorens A, Reig F, Fabra A. 2005. Targeted adriamycin delivery to MXT-B2 metastatic mammary carcinoma cells by transferrin liposomes: effecxt of adriamycin ADR-to lipid ration. Oncol Rep. 14(5):1337-43.

Luce D, Bugel I, Goldberg P, Goldberg M, Salomon C, Billon-Galland M-A, Nicolau J, Quénel, Fevotte J, Brochard P. 2000. Environmental exposure to tremolite and respiratory cancer in New Calidonia: a case-control study. Am J Epidemiol. 151:259-65.

Lund EK, Fairweather-Tait SJ, Wharf SG, Johnson IT. 2001. Chronic exposure to high levels of dietary iron fortification increases lipid peroxidation in the mucosa of the rat large intestine. J Nutr. 131:2928-31.

Lund LG, Aust AE. 1990. Iron mobilization from asbestos by chelators and vitamin C. Arch Biochem Biophys. 278(1):61-4.

——— 1991a. Mobilization of iron from crocidolite asbestos by certain chelators results in enhanced crocidolite-dependent oxygen consumption. Arch Biochem Biophys. 287(1):91-6.

——— 1991b. Iron-catalysed reactions may be responsible for the biochemical and biological effects of asbestos. Biofactors 3:83-9.

——— 1992. Iron mobilization from crocidolite asbestos greatly enhances crocidolite-dependent formation of DNA single-strand breaks in X174 FRI DNA Carcinogenesis 13:637-42.

Lund LG, Williams MG, Dodson RF, Aust AE. 1994. Iron associated with asbestos bodies is responsible for the formation of single strand breaks in phi X174 RFI DNA. Occup Environ Med. 51(3):200-4.

Mader JS, Smyth D, Marshall J, Hoskin DW. 2006. Bovine lactoferricin inhibits basic fibroblast growth factor- and vascular endothelial growth factor 165-induced angiogenesis by competing for heparin-like binding sites on endothelial cells. Am J Pathol. 169(5):1753-66.

Marcus DM, Zinberg N. 1975. Measurement of serum ferritin by radioimmunoassay: results in normal and individuals and patients with breast cancer. J Natl Cancer Inst. 55(4):791-5.

Masini A, Ceccarelli D, Giovannini F, Montosi G, Garuti C, Pietrangelo A. 2000. Iron-induced oxidant streas leads to irreversible mitochondrial dysfunctions and fibrosis in the liver of chronic iron-dosed gerbils. The effect of silybin. J Bioenerg Biomembr. 32(2):175-82.

McDonald JC, McDonald AD. 1996. The epidemiology of mesothelioma in historical context. Eur Respir J. 9:1932-1942.

Mimura J, Fujii-Kuriyama Y. 2003. Functional role of AhR in the expression of toxic effects by TCDD. Biochim Biophys Acta. 1619(3):263-8.

Mistry N, Drobni P, Näslund J, Sunkari VG, Jenssen H, Evander M. 2007. The anti-papillomavirus activity of human and bovine lactoferricin. Antiviral Res. 75(3):258-65.

Mohan KV, Gunasedaran P, Varalakshmi E, Hara Y, Nagini S. 2007. In vitro evaluation of the anticancer effect of lactoferrin and tea polyphenol combination on oral carcinoma cells. Cell Biol Int. 31(6):599-608.

Mohan KV, Letchoumy PV, Hara Y, Nagini S. 2008. Combination chemoprevention of hamster buccal pouch carcinogenesis by bovine milk lactoferrin and black tea polyphenols. Cancer Invest. 26(2):193-201.

Moroz C, Kan M, Chaimof C, Marcus H, Kupfer B, Cuckle HS. 1984. Ferritin-bearing lymphocytes in the diagnosis of breast cancer. Cancer. 54(1):84-9.

Mossman BT, Marsh JP, Shatos MA, Doherty J, Gilbert R, Hill S. 1987. Implication of active oxygen species as second messengers of asbestos toxicity. Drug Chem Toxicol. 10(1-2):157-80.

Mossman BT, Marsh JP, Shatos MA. 1986. Alteration of superoxide dismutase activity in tracheal epithelial cells by asbestos and inhibition of cytotoxicity by antioxidants. Lab Invest. 54(2):204-12.

Mossman BT, Marsh JP. 1989. Evidence supporting a role for active oxygen species in asbestos-induced toxicity and lung disease. Environ Health Perspect. 81:91-4.

Muir AR, Goldberg L. 1961. The tissue response to iron-dextran; an electron-microscope study. J Pathol Bacteriol. 82:471-82.

Nadarajah N, Van Hamme J, Pannu J, Singh A, Ward O. 2002. Enhanced transformation of polycyclic aromatic hydrocarbons using combined Eenton's reagent , microbial treatment and surfactants. Appl Microbiol Biotechnol. 59(4-5):540-4.

Nakase I, Lai H, Singh NP, Sasaki T. 2007.Anticancer properties of artemisinin derivatives and their targeted delivery by trasferrin conjugation. Int J Pharm. [Epub ahead of print]

Nakase M, Inui M, Okumura K, Kamei T, Nakamura S, Tagawa T. 2005. p53 gene therapy of human osteosarcoma using a transferrin-modified cationic liposome. Mol Cancer Ther. 4(4):625-31.

Nelson JM, Stevens RG. 1991. Ferritin-iron increases killing of Chinese hamster ovary cells by x irradiation. Cell Prolif. 24:411.

Nelson RL, Yoo SJ, Tanure JC, Andrianopoulos G, Misumi A. 1989. The effect of iron on experimental colorectal carcinogenesis. Anticancer Res. 9(6):1477-82.

Nelson RL. 2001. Iron and colorectal cancer risk: human studies. 2001. Iron and colorectal cancer risk: human studies. Nutr Rev. 59(5):140-8.

Nicholson WJ, Raffn E. 1995. Recent data on cancer due to asbestos in the U.S.A. and Denmark. Med Lav. 86(5):393-410.

Nishina S, Hino K, Korenage M, Vecchi C, Pietrangelo A, Mizukami Y, Furutani T, Sakai A, Okuda M, Hidaka I, Okita K, Sakaida I. 2008. Hepatitis C virus-induced reactive oxygen species raise hepatic iron level in mice by reducing hepcidin transcription. Gastroenterology. 134(1):226-38.

Norat T, Bingham S, Ferrari P, Slimani N, Jenab M, Mazuir M, Overvod K, Olsen A, Tjønneland A, Clavel F, Boutron-Ruault M-C, Kesse E, Boeing H, Bergmann, MM, Nieters A, Linseisen J, Trichopoulou A, Trichopoulos D, Tountas Y, Berrino F, Palli D, Panico S, Tumino R, Vineis P, Bueno-de-Mesquita HB, Peeters PHM, Engeset D, Lund E, Skeie G, Ardanaz E, González C, Navarro C, Quirós JR, Sanchez M-J, Berglund G, Mattison I, Hallmans G, Palmqvist R, Day NE, Khaw K-T, Key TJ, San Joaquin M, Hémon B, Saracci R, Kaaks R, Riboli E. 2005. Meat, fish, and colorectal cancer risk: The European Prospective Investigation into Cancer and Nutrition. J Natl Cancer Inst. 97:906-16.

Norat T, Lukanova A, Ferrari P, Riboli E. 2002. Meat consumption and colorectal cancer risk: dose-responsive meta-analysis of epidemiological studies. Int J Cancer. 98(2):124-56.

Norat T, Riboli E. 2001. Meat consumption and colorectal cancer: a review of epidemiologic evidence. Nutr Rev. 59(2):37-47.

Oates PS, West AR. 2006. Heme in intestinal epithelial cell turnover, differentiation, detoxification, inflammation, carcinogenesis, absorption and motility. World J Gastroenterol. 12(27):4281-95.

Olynyk JK. 1999. Hepatitis C and iron. Keio J Med. 48(3):124-31.

Olynyk JK, Reddy KR, DiBisceglie AM, Jeffers LJ, Parker TI, Radick JL, Schiff ER, Fujisawa K, Marumo F, Sato C. 1995. Hepatic iron concentration as a predictor of response to interferon alpha therapy in chronic hepatitis C. Gastroenterology. 106(4):1104-9.

Owen RW, Weisgerber UM, Spiegelhalder B, Bartsch H. 1996. Faecal phytic acid and its relation to other putative markers of risk for colorectal cancer. Gut. 38(4):591-7.

Papenhausen PR, Emeson EE, Croft CB, Borowiecki B. 1984. Ferritin-bearing lymphocytes in patients with cancer. Cancer. 53(2):267-71.

Park SH, Aust AE. 1998a. Participation of iron and nitric oxide in the mutagenicity of asbestos in hgprt-, gpt+ Chinese hamster V79 cells. Cancer Res. 58(6):1144-8.

———— 1998b. Regulation of nitric oxide synthase induction by iron and glutathione in asbestos-treated human lung epithelial cells. Arch Biochem Biophys 360(1):47-52.

Pattanapanyasat K, Hoy TG, Jacobs A, Courtney S, Webster DF. 1988. Ferritin-bearing T-lymphocytes and serum ferritin in patients with breast cancer. Br J Cancer. 57(2):193-7.

Peterson DR. 2005. Alcohol, iron-associated oxidative stress, and cancer. Alcohol. 35(3):243-9.

Pierre F, Peiro G, Taché S, Cross AJ, Bingham NG, Gottardi G, Corpet DE, Guéraud F. 2006. New marker of colon cancer risk associated with heme intake: 1,4-dihydroxynonane mercapturic acid. Cancer Epidemiol Biomarkers Prev. 15(11):2274-9.

Pietrangelo A. 2002. Mechanism of iron toxicity. Adv Exp Med Biol. 509:19-43.

———— 2003. Iron-induced oxidant stress in alcoholic liver fibrogenesis. Alcohol. 30(2):121-9.

Pigeon C, Turlin B, Iancu TC, Leroyer P, LeLan J, Deugnier Y, Brissot P, Loréal O. 1999. Carbonyl-iron supplementation induces hepatocyte nuclear changes in BALB/CJ male mice. J Hepatol. 30(5):926-34.

Pike MC, Spicer DV, Dahmoush L, Press MF. 1993. Estrogens, progestogens, normal breast cell proliferation, and breast cancer risk. Epidemiol Rev. 15:17-35.

Piperno A, Sampietro M, D'Alba R, Foffi L, Fargion S, Parma S, Nicoli C, Corbetta N, Pozzi M, Arosio V, Boari G, Fiorelli G. 1996. Iron stores, response to interferon therapy, and effect of iron depletion in chronic hepatitis C. Liver. 16(4):248-54.

Porres JM, Stahl CH, Cheng WH, Fu Y, Roneker KR, Pond WG, Lei XG. 1999. Dietary intrinsic phytate protects colon from lipid peroxidation in pigs with moderately high dietary iron intake. Proc Soc Exp Biol Med. 221(1):80-6.

Porter JB, Huens ER. 1989. The toxic effects of desferrioxamine. Balliere's Clin Haematol. 2:459-74.

Pouzard C, Reelfs O, Kvam E, Tyrrell RM. 1999a. The iron regulatory protein can determine the effectiveness of 5-aminolevulinic acid in inducing protoporphyrin IX in human skin fibroblasts. J Invest Dermatol. 112:419-25.

Pouzard C, Tyrrell RM. 1999. Apoptosis, the role of oxidative stress and the example of solar UV rradiation. Photochem Photobiol. 70:380-90.

Pouzard C, Watkin RD, Brown JE, Tyrrell. 1999b. Ultraviolet radiation induces immediate release of iron in human primary skin fibroblasts: The role of ferritin. Proc Natl Acad Sci USA. 96:6751-6.

Prieto J, Barry M, Sherlock S. 1975. Serum ferritin in patients with iron overload and with acute and chronic liver diseases. Gastroenterology. 68:525-33.

Prutki M, Poljak-Blazi M, Jakopovic M, Tomas D, Stipanci I, Zarkovic N. 2006. Altered iron metabolism, transferrin receptor 1 and ferritin in patients with colon cancer. Cancer Lett. 238(2):188-96.

Pun SH, Tack, F, Bellocq NC, Cheng J, Grubbs BH, Jensen GS, Davis ME, Brewster M, Janicot M, Janssens B, Floren W, Bakker A. 2004. Targeted delivery of RNA-cleaving DNA Enzyme (DNAzyme) to tumor tissue by transferrin-mocified, cyclodextrin-based particles. Cancer Biol and Ther. 3:7641-50.

Purohit V, Russo D, Salin M. 2003. Role of iron in alcoholic liver disease: introduction and summary of the symposium. Alcohol. 30(2):93-7.

Raje D, Mukhtar H, Oshowo A, Ingham Clark C. 2007. What proportion of patients referred to secondary care with iron deficiency anemia have colon cancer: Dis Colon Rectum. 50(8):1211-4.

Rakba N, Loyer P, Gilot D, Delcros JG, Glaise D, Baret PPierre JL, Brissot P, Lescoat G. 2000. Antiproliferative and apoptotic effects of O-Trensox, a new synthetic iron chelator, on differentiated hepatoma cell lines. Carcinogenesis. 21:943-51.

Randerath E, Danna TF, Randernath K. 1992. DNA damage induced by cigarette smoke condensate in vitro as assayed by 32P-postlabeling. Comparison with cigarette smoke-associated DNA adduct profiles in vivo.

Reelfs O, Tyrrell RM, Pourzand C. 2004. Ultraviolet A radiation-immediate iron release is a key modulator of the activation of NF-$_\kappa$B in human skin fibroblasts. 122:1440-7.

Reizenstein P. 1991. Iron, free radicals and cancer. Med Oncol Tumor Pharmacother. 8(4):229-33.

Repine JE, Pfenninger OW. Talmage DW, Berger EM, Pettijohn DE. 1981. Dimethylsulfoxide prevents DNA nicking mediated by ionizing radiation or iron/hydrogen peroxide generated gydroxyl radical. Proc Natl Acad Sci. 78:1001.

Report on Carcinogens. 2002. Iron Dextran Complex. Reasonably anticipated to be a human carcinogen. First listed in the Second Annual Report on Carcinogens (1981).

Rezazadeh H, Athar M. 1997. Evidence that iron-overload promotes 7,12-dimethylbenz(a)anthracene-induced skin tumorigenesis in mice. Redox Rep. 3(5-6):303-9.

Richmond HG. 1959. Induction of sarcoma in the rat by iron-dextran complex. Br Med J. 1(5127):947-49.

———— 1960a. The carcinogenicity of an iron-dextran complex. J Natl Cancer Inst. 24:109-47.

———— 1960b. The carcinogenicity of an iron-dextran complex. Cancer Prog. 1960:24-33.

Robinson CE, Bell DN, Sturdy JH. 1960. Possible association of malignant neoplasm with iron-dextran injection. A case report. Br Med J. 2(5199):648-50.

Roe FJ, Carter RL. 1967. Iron-dextran carcinogenesis in rats: influence of dose on the number and types of neoplasm induced. Int J Cancer. 2(4):370-80.

Roe FJ, Haddow A, Dukes CE, Mitchley BC. 1964. Iron-dextran carcinogenesis in rats: effect of distributing injected material between one, two, four, or six sites. Br J Cancer. 18:801-8.

Roe FJ, Lancester MC. 1964. Natural, metallic and other substances as carcinogens. Br Med Bull. 20:127-33.

Rosen HR, Moroz C, Reiner A, Reinerova M, Stierer M, Svec J, Schemper M, Jakesz R. 1992a. Placental isoferritin associated p43 antigen correlates with reatures of high differentiation in breast cancer. Breast Cancer Res Treat. 24(1):17-26.

Rosen HR, Moroz C, Reiner A, Stierer M, Svec J, Reinerova M, Schemper M, Jakesz R. 1992b. Expression of p43 in breast cancer tissue, correlation with prognostic parameters. Cancer Lett. 67(1):35-45.

Rosen HR, Stierer M, Göttlicher J, Wolf H, Weber R, Vogl E, Eibi M. 1992c. Determination of placental ferritin (PLF)-positive lymphocytes in women in early stages of breast cancer. Int J Cancer. 52(2):229-33.

Rouault TA. 2003. Hepatic iron overload in alcoholic liver disease: why does it occur and what is its role in pathogenesis? Alcohol. 30(2):103-6.

Sadava D, Phillips T. .Lin C, Kane SE. 2002. Transferrin overcomes drug resistance to artemisinin in human small-cell lung carcinoma cells. Cancer Lett. 179(2):151-6.

Saffiotti U, Montesano R, Sellakumar AR, Cefis F, Kaufman DG. 1972. Respiratory tract carcinogenesis induced by different numbers of administrations of benza(á)pyrene and ferric oxide. Cancer Res. 32:1073-81.

Sahoo SK, Labhasetwar V. 2005. Enhanced antiproliferative activity of transferrin-conjugated pacilitaxel-loaded nanoparticles is mediated via sustained intracellular drug retention. Mol Pharm. 2(5):373-83.

Sahu SC, Washington MC. 1991. Iron-mediated oxidative DNA damage detected by fluorometric analysis of DNA unwinding in isolated rat liver nuclei. Biomed Environ Sci. 4(3):219-28.

Sawa T, Akaike T, Kida K, Fukushima Y, Koichi T, Maeda H. 1998. Lipid peroxyl radicals from oxidized oils and heme-iron: implications of a high-fat diet in colon carcinogenesis. Cancer Epidemiol Biomarkers Prev. 7:1007-12.

Schulman I. 1960. Experimental carcinogenesis with iron-dextran. Pediatrics. 26:347-50.

Séité S, Popovic E, Verdier MP, Roguet R, Portes P, Cohen C, Fourtanier A, Galey JB.. 2004. Iron chelation can modulate UVA-induced lipid peroxidation and ferritin expression in human reconstructed epidermis. Photodermatol Photoimmunol Photochem. 20:47-52.

Seitz HK, Stickel R. 2006. Risk factors and mechanisms of hepatocarcinogenesis with special emphasis on alcohol and oxidative stress. Biol Chem. 387(4):349-60.

Selby JV, Friedmann GD. 1988. Epidemiological evidence of an association of body iron stores and risk of cancer. Int J Cancer. 41:677.

Senesse P, Meance S, Cottet V, Faivre J, Boutron-Ruault MC. 2004. High dietary iron and copper: a case control study in Burgundy, France.

Nutr Cancer. 49(1):66-71.

Seril DN, Liao J, Yang GY, Yang CS. 2003. Oxidative stress and ulcerative colitis-associated carcinogenesis: studies in humans and animal models. Carcinogenesis. 24(3):353-62.

Sesnik ALA, Termont DSML, Kleibeuker JH, Van der Meer R. 1999. Red meat and colon cancer: the cytotoxic and hyperproliferative effects of dietary heme. 1999. Cancer Res. 59:5704-9.

Shan Y, Lambrecht RW, Bonkovsky HL. 2005. Association of hepatitis C virus infection with serum iron status: analysis of data from the third National Health and Nutrition Examination Survey. Clin Infect Dis. 40(6):834-41.

Sharma JB, Jain S, Mallika V, et al. 2004. A prospective, partially randomized study of pregnancy outcomes and hematologic responses to oral and intramuscular iron treatment in moderately anemic pregnant women. Am J Clin Nutr. 79:116-22.

Shatos MA, Doherty JM, Marsh JP, Mossman BT. 1987. Prevention of asbestos-induced cell death in rat lung fibroblasts and alveolar macrophages by scavengers of active oxygen species. Environ Res. 44(1):103-16.

Shen HM, Ong CN, Shi CY. 1995. Involvement of reactive oxygen species in aflatoxin B1-induced cell injury in cultured rat hepatocytes. Toxicology. 99(1-2):115-23.

Shen Z, Bosbach D, Hochella MF Jr, Bish DL, Williams MG Jr, Dodson RF, Aust AE. 2000. Using in vitro iron deposition on asbestos to model asbestos bodies formed in human lung. Chem Res Toxicol. 13(9):913-21.

Shimamura M, Yamamoto Y, Ashino H, Oikawa T, Hazato T, Tsuda H, Iigo M. 2004. Bovine lactoferrin inhibits tumor-induced angiogenesis. Int J Cancer. 111(1):111-6.

Shimida T, Fujji-Kuriyama T. 2004. Metabolic activation of polycyclic aromatic hydrocarbons to carcinogens by cytochromes P450 1A1 and 1B1. Cancer Sci. 95:1-6.

Shimida T. 2006. Xenobiotic-metabolizing enzymes involved in activation and detoxification of carcinogenic polycyclic aromatic hydrocarbons. Drug Metab Pharmacokinet. 21(4):257-76.

Shterman N, Kupfer B, Moroz C. 1991. Comparison of transferrin receptors, iron content and isoferritin profile in normal and malignant human breast cell lines. Pathobiology. 59(1):19-25.

Simonart T, Boelaert JR, Andrei G, van den Oord JJ, Degraef C, Hermans P, Noel JC, Van Vooren JP, Heenen M, De Clercq E, Snoeck R. 2002. Desferrioxamine enhances AISA-associated Kaposi's sarcoma tumor development in a xenograft model. Int J Cancer. 100:140-3.

Singh S, Khodr H, Taylor M, Hider RC. 1995. Therapeutic iron chelators and their potential side-effects. Biochem Soc Symp. 61:127-37.

Smith KR, Aust AE. 1997. Mobilization of iron from urban particulates leads to generation of reactive oxygen species in vitro and induction of ferritin synthesis in human lung epithelial cells. Chem Res Toxicol. 10(7):828-34.

Smith KR, Vernath JM, Hu AA, Lighty JS, Aust AE. 2000. Interleukin-8 levels in human lung epithelial cells are increased in response to coal fly ash and vary with bioavailability of iron, as a function of particle size and source of coal. Chem Res Toxicol. 13(2):118-25.

Solomons NW, Schümann K. 2004. Intramuscular administration of iron dextran is inappropriate for treatment of moderate pregnancy anemia, both in intervention research on underprivileged women and in routine prenatal care provided by public health services. Am J Clin Nutr. 79(1):1-3.

Stål P, Johansson I, Ingelman-Sundberg M, Hagen K, Hultcrantz R. 1996. Hepatotoxicity induced by iron overload and alcohol. Studies on the role of chelatable iron, cytochromes P450 2E1 and lipid peroxidation. J Hepatol. 25(4)"538-46.

Stål P. 1995. Iron as a hepatotoxin. Dig Dis. 13(4):205-22.

Stevens RG, Beasley RP, Blumberg BS. 1986. Iron-binding proteins and risk of cancer in Taiwan. J Natl Cancer Inst. 76(4):605-10.

Stevens RG, Graubard BI, Micozzi MS, Neriishi K, Blumberg BS. 1994. Moderate elevation of body iron level and increased risk of cancer occurrence and death. Int J Cancer. 56(3)364-9.

Stevens RG, Jones DY, Micozzi MS, Taylor PR. 1988. Body iron stores and the risk of cancer. N Engl J Med.319:1047-52.

Stevens RG, Kalkwarf DR. 1990. Iron, radiation, and cancer. Env Health Persp. 87:291-300.

Stevens RG, Morris JE, Anderson LE. 2000. Hemochromatosis heterozygotes may constitute a radiation-sensitive subpopulation. Radiat Res. 153(6):844-7.

Stevens RG. 1990. Iron and the risk of cancer. Med Oncol Tumor Pharmacother. 7(2-3):177-81.

———— 1991. Dietary effects on breast cancer. Lancet. 338(8760):186-7.

———— 1992. Iron and cancer. In: *Iron and Human Disease.* Lauffer RB, ed. Boca Raton: CRC Press, pp 333-47.

Stone WL, Papas AM, LeClair IO, Qui M, Ponder T. 2002. The influence of dietary iron and tocopherols on oxidative stress and ras-p21 levels in the colon. Cancer Detect Prev. 26(1):78-84.

Sumida Y, Kanemasa K, Fukumoto K, Yoshida N, Sakai K. 2007. Effects of dietary iron reduction versus phlebotomy in patients with chronic hepatitis C: results from a randomized, controlled trial on 40 Japanese patients. Intern Med. 46(10):637-42.

Sun-Hee P, Aust AE. 1998. Participation of iron and nitric oxide in mutagenicity of asbestos in hgprt-, gpt+ Chinese hamster V79 cells. Cancer Res. 58:1144-48.

Sutnik AJ, Blumberg BS, Lustbader ED. 1974. Elevated serum iron levels and persistent Australian antigen (HBsAg). Ann Intern Med. 81:855-6.

Suzuki Y, Saito H, Suzuki M, Hosoki Y, Sakurai S, Fujimoto Y, Kohgo Y. 2002. Up-regulation of transferrin receptor expression in hepatocytes by habitual alcohol drinking is implicated in hepatic iron overload in alcoholic liver disease. Alcohol Clin Exp Res. 26(8 Suppl): 265-315.

Swanson CA. 2003. Iron intake and regulation: implications for iron deficiency and iron overload. Alcohol. 30(2):99-102.

Talley NJ, Chute CG, Larson DE, Epstein R, Lydick EG, Melton LJ 3rd. 1989. Risk for colorectal adenocarcinoma in pernicious anemia. A population-based cohort study. Ann Intern Med. 111(9):738-42.

Thedering F. 1964. The tolerance of iron therapy with special reference to the carcinogenic effect of the dextran-iron complex. Med Welt. 17:277-82.

Tsuda H, Sekine K, Fujita K, Ligo M. 2002. Cancer prevention by bovine lactoferrin and underlying mechanisms – a review of experimental and clinical studies. Biochem Cell Biol. 80(1):131-6.

Tsuda H, Sekine K, Ushida Y, Kuhara T, Takasuka N, Iigo M, Han BS, Moore MA. 2000. Milk and dairy products in cancer prevention: focus on bovine lactoferrin. Mutat Res. 462(2-3):227-33.

Tsuda H, Sekine K. 2000. Milk components as cancer chemopreventive agents. Asian Pac J Cancer Prev. 1(4):277-82.

Turlin B, Deugnier Y. 2002. Iron overload disorders. Clin Liver Dis. 6(2):481-96.

Turner HM, Grace HG. 1938. An investigation into cancer mortality among males in certain Sheffield trades. J Hyg 38:90-103.

Turver CJ, Brown RC. 1987. The role of catalytic iron in asbestos induced lipid peroxidation and DNA-strand breakage in C3H10T1/2 cells. Br

J Cancer. 56(2):133-6.

Tyrrell RM. 1991. UVA (320-380 nm) radiation as an oxidative stress. In: Sies H, ed. *Oxidative Stress: Oxidants and Antioxidants*. London: Academic Press, pp 57-83.

———— 1996. Activation of mammalian gene expression by the UV component of sunlight – from models to reality. Bioassays. 18:139-48.

Ulbrich EJ, Lebrecht A, Schneider I, Ludwig E, Koelbl H, Hefler LA. 2003. Serum parameters of iron metabolism in patients with breast cancer. Anticancer Res. 23(6D):5107-9.

Valenti L, Pulixi EA, Arosio P, Cremonesi L, Biasiotto G, Dongiovanni P, Maggioni M, Fargion S, Fracanzani AL. 2007. Relative contribution of iron genes, dysmetabolism and hepatitis C virus (HCV)in the pathogenesis of altered iron regulation in HCV chronic hepatitis. Haematologica 92(8):1037-42.

Valko M, Morris H, Mazúr M, Rapta P, Bilton RF. 2001. Oxygen free radical generating mechanisms in the colon: do the semiquinones of vitamin K play a role in the aetology of colon cancer? Biochim Biophys Acta. 1527(3):161-6.

Valko M, Rhodes CJ, Moncol J, Izakovic M, Mazur M. 2006. Free radicals, metals and antioxidants in oxidative stress-induced cancer. Chem Biol Interact. 160(1):1-40.

Vallier J, Rebouillat M. 1962. [Research on the in vivo carcinogenic activity of an iron-dextran complex in the rat.] CR Seances Soc Biol Fil. 156:691-93. (French)

van Maanen JM, Borm Pj, Knaapen A, van Herwijnen M, Schilderman PA, Smith KR, Aust AE, Tomatis M, Fubini B. 1999. In vitro effects of coal fly ashes: hydroxyl radical generation, iron release, and DNA damage and toxicity in rat lung epithelial cells. Inhal Toxicol. 11(12):1123-41.

Van Thiel DH, Friedlander L, Faginoli S, Wright HI, Irish W, Gavaler JS. 1994. Response to interferon á therapy is influenced by the iron content of the liver. J Hepatol. 20:410-5.

Vandewalle B, Granier AM, Peyrat JP, Bonneterre J, Lefebvre J. 1985. Transferrin receptors in cultured breast cancer cells. J Cancer Res Clin Oncol. 110(1):71-6.

Varadhachary A, Wolf JS, Petrak K, O'Malley BW Jr, Spadaro M, Curcio C, Forni G, Pericle F. 2004. Oral lactoferrin inhibits growth of established tumors and potentiates conventional chemotherapy. Int J Cancer. 111(3):398-403.

Vile GF, Tanew-Ilitschew A, Tyrell RM. 1995. Activation of NF-kappa

B in human skin fibroblasts by the oxidative stress generated by UVA radiation. Photochem Photobiol. 62:463-8.

Vile GF, Tyrrell RM. 1995. UVA radiation-induced oxidative damage to lipids and proteins in vitro and in human skin fibroblasts is dependent on iron and singlet oxygen. Free Radic Biol Med. 18:721-30.

Vrbanec D, Petriceviæ B. 2007. Estrogen and progesterone receptor status in primary breast cancer – a study of 11,273 patients from the year 1990-2002. Coll Antropol. 31(2):535-40.

Ward PP, Paz E, Conneely OM. 2005. Multifunctional roles of lactoferrin: a critical overview. Cell Mol Life Sci. 62(22):2540-8.

Warheit DB, Hill LH, Brody AR. 1984. In vitro effects of crocidolite asbestos and wollastonite on pulmonary macrophages and serum complement. Scan Electron Microsc. (Pt 2):919-26.

Weinberg ED. 1981. Iron and neoplasia. Biol Trace Elem Res. 3:55-80.

———— 1984. Iron withholding: a defence against infection and neoplasia. Physiol Rev. 64:65-102.

———— 1989. Iron, asbestos, and carcinogenicity. Lancet. 1:1399-40.

———— 1992a. Roles of iron in neoplasia: promotion, prevention and therapy. Biol Trace Elem Res. 34:123-40.

———— 1992b. Iron depletion: a defence against intracellular infection and neoplasia. Life Sci. 50:1289-97.

———— 1993. Association of iron with respiratory tract neoplasia. J Trace Elem Exp Med. 6:117-23.

———— 1994. Role of iron in colorectal cancer. BioMetals. 7:211-6.

———— 1996. Iron withholding: a defense against viral infections. BioMetals. 9:393-9.

———— 1996a. The role of iron in cancer. Euro J Cancer Prev. 5:19-36.

———— 2001. Lung cancer among industrial sand workers exposed to crystalline silica. Am J Epidemiology. 154(3):288.

———— 2002. Therapeutic potential of human transferrin and lactoferrin. ASM News. 68(2):65-69.

———— 2005. Iron withholding as a defense against disease. In: Weiss G, Gordeuk VR, Hershko, eds. 2005. *Anemia of Chronic Disease*. Boca Raton: Taylor and Francis.

Weinberg ED. 2007. Antibiotic properties and applications of lactoferrin. Current Pharm Design. 13:801-11.

Weinstein RE, Bond BH, Silberberg BK, Vaughn CB, Subbaiah P, Pieper DR. 1989. Tissue ferritin concentration and prognosis in carcinoma of the breast. Breast Cancer Res Treat. 14(3):349-53.

Weiss G, Gordeuk VR, Hershko, eds. 2005. *Anemia of Chronic Disease*. Boca Raton: Taylor and Francis.

Weitzman SA, Graceffa P. 1984. Asbestos catalyzes hydroxyl and superoxide radical generation from hydrogen peroxide. Arch Biochem Biophys. 228(1):373-6.

Weizer-Stern O, Adamsky K, Margalit O, Ashur-Favian O, Givol D, Amariglio N, Rechavi G. 2007. Hepcidin, a key regulator of iron metabolism, is transcriptionally activated by p53. Br J Haematol. 138(2):253-62.

Whiting RF, Wei L, Stitch HF. 1981. Chromosome-damaging activity of ferritin and its relation to chelation and reduction of iron. Cancer Res. 41:1628.

Wolf JS, Li G, Varadhachary A, Petrak K, Schneyer M, Li D, Ongkasuwan J, Zhang X, Taylor RJ, Strome SE, O'Malley BW Jr. 2007. Oral lactoferrin results in T cell-dependent tumor inhibition of head and neck squamous cell carcinoma in vivo. Clin Cancer Res. 13(5):1601-10.

Wright A, Donaldson K, Davis JM. 1983. Cytotoxic effect of asbestos on macrophages in different activation states. 51:109-17.

Wurzelmann JI, Silver A, Schreinemachers DM, Sandler RS, Everson RB. 1996. Iron intake and the risk of colorectal cancer. Cancer Epidemiol Biomarkers and Prev. 5:503-7.

Wyllie S, Liehr JG. 1997. Release of iron from ferritin storage by redox cycling of stilbene and steroid estrogen metabolites: a mechanism of induction of free radical damage by estrogen. Arch Biochem Biophys. 346(2):180-6.

Xiong S, She H, Sung CK, Tsukamoto H. 2003. Iron-dependent activation of NF-kappaB in Kuppfer cells: a priming mechanism for alcoholic liver disease. Alcohol. 30(2):107-13.

Xu A, Wu LJ, Santella RM, Hei TK. 1999. Role of oxyradicals in mutagenicity and DNA damage induced by crocidolite asbestos in mammalian cells. Cancer Res. 59(23):5922-6.

Xu A, Zhou H, Yu DZ, Hei TK. 2002. Mechanisms of the genotoxicity of crocidolite asbestos in mammalian cells: implication from mutation patterns by reactive oxygen species. Environ Health Perspect. 110(10):1003-8.

Xue W, Warshawsky D. 2005. Metabolic activation of polycyclic and heterocyclic aromatic hydrocarbons and DNA damage: a review. Toxicol

Appl Pharmacol. 206(1):73-93.

Yamauchi K, Wakabayashi H, Shin K, Takase M. 2006. Bovine lacto-ferrin: benefits and mechanisms of action against infections. Biochem Cell Biol. 84(3):291-6.   '

Yiakouvaki A, Savovic J, Al-Quenaei A, Dowden J, Pourzand C. 2006. Caged-iron chelators a novel approach towards protecting skin cells against UVA-induced necrotic cell death. J Invest Dermatol. 126:2287-95.

Yu Z, Eaton JW, Persson HL. 2003. The radioprotective agent, amifos-tine, suppresses the reactivity of intralysosomal iron. 8(6):347-55.

Zhong JL, Yiakouvaki A, Patricia H, Tyrrell RM, Pourzand. 2004. Susceptibility of skin cells to UVA-induced necrotic cell death reflects the intracellular level of labile iron. J Invest Dermatol. 123:771-80.

Chapter 7

Additional Iron-Deposition Diseases

Introduction

We have discussed the neurotoxicology and carcinogenicity of iron in some detail. In all probability, all diseases of aging are either caused or exacerbated by the high body iron burden that exists among aging people in North America (Zacharaski et al. 2000, Fleming et al. 2002). In this chapter, we will explore iron toxicology as it relates to several diseases or circumstances:

- **Hereditary hemochromatosis**
- **Cardiovascular diseases**
- **Adult-onset diabetes**
- **Arthritis**
- **Osteoporosis**
- **Stroke**
- **Traumatic brain injury**
- **Hearing loss**
- **Age-related eye diseases**
- **Thalassemia**
- **Pituitary gland toxicity**
- **Reproductive organ damage**
- **Renal toxicity**
- **Porphyria cutanea tarda**
- **Sudden infant death syndrome**
- **Endurance athletics**

For the sake of brevity, although a considerable body of evidence may link each of these illnesses to iron excess, only the most germane references are cited.

Hereditary Hemochromatosis

The most common form of iron overload disease is an inherited condition, hereditary hemochromatosis. The gene responsible is known as the *HFE* gene. Two gene mutations, referred to as C282Y and H63D, are the most common types, occurring in one out of 200-400 Caucasians. About 85% of patients with hemochromatosis are homozygous for the C282Y mutation, which results in abnormal absorption of iron. Weinberg states (Garrison, ed. 2005, p 8):

> Normally the body employs various sophisticated maneuvers to regulate the amount of iron absorbed. The total amount of body iron in healthy adults is maintained at a level of about 4 grams, which is distributed in proteins and serum. The daily 1-2 mg of iron absorbed from diet is prudently balanced by daily excretion in perspiration, urine, and feces of 1-2 mg.
>
> In hemochromatosis patients, however, the daily amount of iron absorbed is 2-4 mg, but the daily excretion remains unchanged. Accordingly, were the imbalance to begin in a 20-year-old person, about 1 gram/year would be accumulated and would need to be hidden away in innocuous packages throughout the various organs. By the time that 10-15 grams have accumulated, clinical symptoms in one or more organs might have begun to appear. Untreated, some hereditary hemochromatosis patients have been reported to collect as much as 50 grams during their lifetime.

The clinical symptoms of hereditary hemochromatosis include diabetes, extreme fatigue, joint pain, sexual dysfunction (impotence and others), skin bronzing, heart fluttering, depression, and abdominal pain (Garrison, ed. 2005, p 9).

Cardiovascular Diseases

In 1981, Jerome Sullivan of the Veterans Affairs Medical Center, Charleston, South Carolina hypothesized that the North American epidemic of heart disease is due to excessive amounts of iron. From then until the end of the 20th century, the "iron theory of heart disease" was a subject of great controversy. Today, we know for certain that iron excess is involved in the continuing epidemic of heart disease. However, we don't yet know all of the various ways that iron is involved. Several mechanisms by which iron excess damages the cardiovascular system include:

1. Iron is deposited in atherosclerotic lesions where redox cycles, producing oxidized lipids (LDL-oxidation).
2. Iron is directly toxic to the heart muscle, causing muscle weakness as observed in hemochromatotics and thalassemics.
3. Iron interferes with electrical functions of the heart, resulting in "heart flutters," also as seen in hemochromatotics and thalassemics.

Iron Deposits are Found in Atherosclerotic Lesions

The fact that iron is found in atherosclerotic lesions is well established, and has been known since 1944 when Blumenthal et al. (1944) analyzed calcification associated with atherosclerotic plaques. Many subsequent studies have confirmed this early report. In the 1960s, the World Health Organization defined atherosclerosis as follows: "Atherosclerosis is a variable combination of changes of the intima of arteries (as distinct from arterioles) consisting of the focal accumulation of lipids, complex carbohydrates, blood and blood products, fibrous tissue and calcium deposits, and associated with medial changes."

Attention recently has been refocused on iron deposits in atherosclerotic lesions by Chau (2000), who stated, "Recently, studies conducted in our laboratory and others have demonstrated iron deposition is prominent in human atherosclerosis. The iron deposits appear to colocalize with ceroid, an end product of extensively oxidized lipid and protein complex, in lesions, providing histological evidence to support the iron hypothesis."

Many studies have identified oxidation of LDL-cholesterol by iron in atherosclerotic lesions (Reviewed by Brewer 2007). There seems to be little doubt that iron that is contained within atherosclerotic plaques oxidizes LDL-cholesterol and, in that way, contributes to atherosclerosis and coronary artery disease.

Iron is Directly Cardiotoxic

Terminology associated with the term, "heart disease:"

- **Atherosclerosis**: the loss of pliability of arteries ("hardening of the arteries") where many parts of the arterial system are affected by cholesterol-laden concretions of minerals, dead red blood cells, cholesterol, and oxidized lipids.
- **Ischemic heart disease:** Lack of blood flow to the heart resulting in a lack of oxygen to support proper heart function. There are at least three well-known causes of ischemic heart disease (there may be other causes, but these are the most common):
    o **Coronary artery disease** refers to narrowing of the coronary artery resulting from atherosclerotic lesions that may result in insufficient delivery of blood to the heart—one form of ischemic heart disease.
    o **Cardiomyopathy** is the weakening of heart muscle that is conspicuous in hereditary hemochromatosis and thalassemia. Heart muscle is very sensitive to iron's toxic effects due, in part, to a high rate of metabolism that has a requirement for ready oxygen supply. Oxygen radicals generated under the influence of excess (or "free") iron weaken heart muscle.
    o **Cardiac arrhythmias** are irregular heartbeats. The beating of the heart is controlled by electrical impulses. Although cardiac arrhythmias are not always due to iron overload, iron overload as illustrated by hemochromatosis and thalassemia does lead to cardiac arrhythmias.

Ischemic heart disease may be a consequence of coronary artery disease, but coronary artery disease is not always the cause of ischemic heart disease. Accumulation of iron in heart muscle is directly cardiotoxic. Many cases of ischemic heart disease are due to cardiomyopathy or cardiac arrhythmias resulting from cardiotoxicity of iron, rather than from lack of blood supply due to constriction of the coronary artery.

It is interesting that people with hereditary hemochromatosis are not particularly prone to atherosclerosis. Instead, hemochromatotics are more prone to develop cardiomyopathy and/or cardiac arrhythmias. Both heart muscles and electrical activity of the heart are significantly modified in hemochromatotics and thassalemics.

One reason that hereditary hemochromatosis does not lead to atherosclerosis is thought to be because their macrophages are deficient in iron. Macrophages use redox cycling of iron/oxygen to kill invading organisms and to scavenge dead tissue. By scavenging dying cells at sites where atherosclerotic plaques are forming, macrophages actually contribute to formation of plaques. In hemochromatotics, this function is suppressed. Thus, instead of developing atherosclerosis, iron targets heart muscle and heart electrical activity, causing cardiomyopathy and cardiac arrhythmias.

Epidemiology

A role for iron in heart disease risk was first proposed by Sullivan (1981). He based his hypothesis on the male/female difference in incidence. Males are much more severely afflicted than females prior to menopause, but the difference changes in postmenopausal women. By age 60 or 70, death from heart disease is approximately the same for men and women. Sullivan argued that women of childbearing age loose blood on a monthly basis and are thereby protected from iron excess.

The role of iron in heart diseases has been studied more than any of the other diseases of aging covered in this review. Even though volumes have been written on the role of iron in hereditary hemochromatosis, cancer, and thalassemia, no other aspect of iron toxicology has received as much public attention as has the role of iron in heart diseases (and cardiovascular diseases in general). The conflicting results of epidemiological studies have met with fierce debates and have received a great deal of public attention. Headline articles have been published in magazines like *McLean's*, *Time*, and the *Wall-Street Journal*.

For instance, Victor Herbert (1994) of the Hematology and Nutrition Laboratory Veteran's Affairs and Mount Sinai Medical Centers wrote a Letter to the Editor of the American Journal of Clinical Nutrition in response to a study that was supposed to have refuted the "iron hypothesis of heart disease:" The study was publicized by an article in the *Wall Street Journal*, "U.S. Study Questions Link of Heart Disease to Body's Iron Level". This is Herbert's response:

Iron worsens high-cholesterol-related coronary artery disease.

Dear Sir:

Misled by a November 11, 1993 headline and press release from the American Heart Association "Round 2: Autopsy Study Appears to Refute Link of Excess Iron to Heart Disease Risk," the *Wall Street Journal* on November 12, 1993 published an equally misleading story under the equally misleading title, "U.S. Study Questions Link of Heart Disease to Body's Iron Level."

Herbert went on to defend the hypothesis that high iron stores cause oxidation of LDL-cholesterol, which is involved in atherogenesis.

By 1996, it became nearly impossible to keep up with the vast numbers of epidemiological studies regarding a possible role for iron in cardiovascular diseases. Meyers (1996) reported, "At least seven epidemiologic studies have found a positive association between coronary heart disease and several indicators of body iron. Conversely, 18 epidemiological studies have shown a negative or no association. While biochemically appealing, the iron hypothesis remains unproven."

We will not go into detail in this book on the "iron hypothesis of heart disease." Instead, we direct the interested reader to basic literature.

Books and Articles

- Lauffer RB. 1993. *Iron and Your Heart*. New York: St Martin's Press.
- Facchini FS. 2002. *The Iron Factor of Aging. Why Do Americans Age Faster?* Tucson: Fenestra Books.
- Garrison, ed. 2005. *Exposing the Hidden Dangers of Iron*. By Weinberg ED. Nashville: Cumberland House.
- Sullivan JL. 1992. Stored iron as a risk factor for ischemic heart disease. In: Lauffer RB, ed. *Iron and Human Disease*. Boca Raton, Ann Arbor, London, Tokyo: CRC Press.

Ferritin Light Chain

Iron is definitely involved in heart disease, but its actual role is not yet completely understood. There is ample and undeniable evidence that LDL-cholesterol oxidation resulting from redox cycling of iron is involved (See references above).

An interesting new approach to defining the role of iron in atherosclerosis was reported by You et al. (2003). The approach is referred as "proteomic analysis." You and coworkers define proteomics as follows: "The approach we employed was proteomics, the analysis of a proteome, which can detect proteins that are associated with a disease by measuring their levels of expression between control and disease states. To our knowledge, this is the first application of proteomics to study coronary artery disease." Ferritin is composed of two subunits, designated H (heavy) and L (light) chains. It was demonstrated that the ferritin light chain in coronary arteries is significantly increased in patients with coronary artery disease.

Excess Iron is Characteristic of Type 2 Diabetes

Our discussion of the relationship between body iron burden and type 2 diabetes proceeds along three lines:

1. Experimental studies on iron overload in laboratory animals.
2. Frequency of type 2 diabetes in hereditary hemochromatosis

and thalassemia.

3. Elevated serum ferritin in type 2 diabetes.

Iron Overload in Laboratory Animals Results in Diabetes

Studies of iron-loaded rats demonstrate the deposition of iron in liver, pancreas, spleen, heart, pituitary gland, and kidney (Whittaker et al. 1996; Vayenas et al. 1998; Chua-anusorn et al. 1999; Pereira et al. 1999; Papanastasiou et al. 2000). Cardiomyopathy, cardiac arrhythmias, and loss of pancreatic function occur. Iron-loaded rats rapidly lose pancreatic function and become diabetic.

Type 2 Diabetes in HHC and Thalassemia

Hereditary hemochromatosis and ß-thalassemia are two well-known conditions that lead to iron overload. People with hereditary hemochromatosis absorb excessive amounts of iron and become overloaded. In the thalassemias, blood transfusion results in iron overload. Iron deposits in the pancreas are generally found, and diabetes is common in both conditions.

Elevated Serum Ferritin in Type 2 Diabetes

The role for iron in type 2 diabetes is exceptionally well-documented. Extensive iron stores can cause type 2 diabetes among people with hereditary hemochromatosis (Witte et al. 1996). It has been hypothesized that formation of hydroxyl radicals catalyzed by iron contributes initially to insulin resistance, subsequently to decreased insulin secretion, and then to the development of type 2 diabetes (Andrews 1999). The literature is replete with articles on this topic, and there is general agreement that high body iron burden as indicated by elevated serum ferritin is a risk factor for type 2 diabetes.

A recent publication summarizes current knowledge of the relationship between high iron stores and type 2 diabetes. "Body iron stores in relation to risk of type 2 diabetes in apparently healthy women" (Jiang et al. 2004):

> Type 2 diabetes is a common manifestation of hemochromatosis, a disease of iron overload. However, it is not clear whether

higher iron stores predict the development of type 2 diabetes in a healthy population. The objective of this study is to examine plasma ferritin concentration and the ratio of the concentrations of transferrin receptors to ferritin in relation to type 2 diabetes.

This was a prospective nested case-control study within the Nurses' Health Study cohort. Of 32,826 women who provided blood samples during 1989-1990 and were free of diagnosed diabetes, cardiovascular disease, and cancer, 698 developed diabetes during 10 years of follow-up. The 716 controls were matched to cases on age, race, and fasting status; and on body mass index (BMI) for cases in the top BMI decile. Among cases, the mean concentration of ferritin was significantly higher (109[105] vs 71.5 [68.7] ng/ml for controls; P=.01 for the difference, and the mean (SD) ratio of tranferrin receptors to ferritin was significantly lower (102[205] vs 102 [205] vs 141 [340], respectively, P=.01).... Conclusions: Higher iron stores (reflected by an elevated ferritin concentration and a lower ratio of transferrin receptors to ferritin) are associated with an increased risk of type 2 diabetics in healthy women independent of known diabetes risk factors.

Iron and Arthritis

Arthritis is one of the key markers for hereditary hemochromatosis (HHC). The arthritis of hereditary hemochromatosis has been described in the *Iron Disorders Institute Guide to Hemochromatosis* (Garrison, ed. 2001, pp 109-110):

> Pain or aching in joints of hands, especially the first two metacarpal phalanges (knuckles), hips, knees, and ankles are most commonly associated with iron overload. Joint aches or arthralgia is the single most common clinical feature for patients with HHC. Joint pain is very common in the population and hence not specific, but aching of the ankles or of the knuckles and first joint of the second and third fingers (called iron fist) is an unusual pattern that should suggest HHC."
>
> These same hand joints are also often involved in rheumatoid arthritis, but, in hemochromatosis/iron overload-related arthritis, the patient will usually test negative in the blood for rheumatoid factor....Arthritis in iron overload is

commonly misdiagnosed as seronegative rheumatoid arthritis, osteoarthritis, or gout."

Iron Overload Causes Osteoporosis

A number of iron-overload conditions are known to result in osteo-porosis and osteopenia. For instance, in a set of 38 untreated HFE-related hemochromatotic patients, 79% were osteopenic and 34% osteoporotic (Guggenbuhl et al. 2005). Blood transfusions are given to treat several hereditary blood illnesses such as sickle cell anemia and thalassemia. In a group of 18 transfused thalassemic children, 61% had low bone mass (Vogiatzi et al. 2004). Osteoporosis also accompanies African siderosis. For a review of the osteoporosis of iron overload, refer to "Iron loading: a risk factor for osteoporosis." (Weinberg 2006.)

Because known iron-overload conditions result in an increased incidence of osteoporosis, the next question to be answered is, "What proportion of people with osteoporosis have iron overload disease?"

Stroke and Traumatic Brain Injury

Stroke, also referred to as cerebrovascular insufficiency, is a major cause of morbidity and mortality in our society today. Each year more than 1 million people in the U.S. alone are subjected to stroke. Traumatic brain injury is in many respects similar to stroke because, in both circumstances, blood is lost through the vasculature that feeds the brain. In both stroke and traumatic brain injury, an increased body burden of iron increases the danger of oxidative damage to the brain (Terada et al. 1992; Chang et al. 2005).

Elevated Serum Ferritin is a Risk Factor for Stroke

The relationship between iron and stroke has been known for many years. Tarada et al. (1992, p 314) stated: "Great interest has emerged recently in the potential role of iron in the genesis of cere-brovascular diseases. In stroke syndromes, the brain appears to be particularly sensitive to iron-mediated oxidative damage because of its high levels of polyunsaturated lipids, which are vital for neural transmission, its acidic environment during ischemia, and its high metabolic rate. The ability of excess iron to facilitate peroxidation of brain lipids has been amply demonstrated."

Erdemoglu and Ozbakir (2002) designed a prospective study to determine whether increased ferritin levels might help estimate the severity of prognosis of stroke. Fifty-one patients with a diagnosis of acute stroke were included in the study within 24 hours from onset of symptoms. Conclusions: "Increased serum ferritin levels correlate to severity of stroke and the size of the lesion."

van der A et al. (2005) wrote an article entitled, "Serum ferritin is a risk factor for stroke in postmenopausal women." The authors studied the association between iron status and stroke risk in a population-based cohort of 11,471 Dutch postmenopausal women between 49 and 70 years of age. Women were included between 1993 and 1997 and followed up until January 1, 2000 for cerebrovascular events. Serum ferritin, serum iron, and transferrin saturation were measured as markers of iron status. Conclusions: "Neither serum iron nor transferrin saturation was associated with an increased stroke risk. However, higher serum ferritin concentrations in postmenopausal women are associated with an increased risk of ischemic stroke."

Increased Body Iron Burden in Traumatic Brain Injury

Millan et al. (2007) investigated "whether high serum ferritin levels, as an index of increased cellular iron stores, are associated with poor outcome, hemorrhagic transformation, and brain edema after treatment with tissue plasminogen activator in patients with acute ischemic stroke" Conclusions: "Increased body iron stores are associated with poor outcome, symptomatic hemorrhagic transformation, and severe edema in patients treated with plasminogen activator after ischemic stroke. These findings suggest that iron overload may offset the beneficial effect of thrombolytic therapies."

In a review article, Hua et al. (2007) reported on the toxicity of iron and thrombin in brain injury after intracerebral hemorrhage.

"Recent studies have helped to elucidate the mechanisms that trigger pathophysiological changes in and around hematoma." In particular, they have focused attention on the role of thrombin and iron, released upon red blood cell lysis as two major factors causing brain injury after intracerebral hemorrhage.

What is the Role of Iron in Hearing Loss?

This portion of our story begins in rather strange territory—hearing loss induced by some antibiotics. The fact that gentamicin induces hearing loss has been known for many years, but it was not until 1997 that the cause for this hearing loss became better understood. Song et al. (1997) published the first article to shed light on the role of iron in gentamicin-induced hearing loss. The article title was, "Protection from gentamicin ototoxicity by iron chelators in guinea pig *in vivo*." Conclusions: "These results confirm that iron and free radicals play a crucial role in the toxic side effects of gentamicin. Furthermore, they suggest that iron chelators, which are well-established drugs in clinical therapy, may be promising therapeutic agents to reduce aminoglycoside ototoxicity."

A number of studies quickly confirmed that iron chelators are able to decrease the ototoxicity of aminoglycoside antibiotics (Song et al. 1998; Conlon et al. 1998; Chen et al. 1999; Bates 2003; Lautermann et al. 2004).

Conlon et al. (1998) studied the mechanism involved in neomycin/iron-induced hearing loss:

> Increasing evidence suggests that aminoglycosides ototoxicity is mediated by the formation of an aminoglycoside-iron complex and that the creation of this complex is a preliminary step in generation of free radical species and subsequent hair cell death. In this study, we have assessed the ability of the iron chelator deferoxamine to attenuate the hearing loss induced by an ototoxic dose of the aminoglycoside, neomycin.... These results provide further evidence of the intrinsic role of iron in aminoglycoside ototoxicity and suggest that desferoxamine may have a therapeutic role in attenuating the cytotoxic action

of aminoglycoside antibiotics.

Yamasoba et al. (1999) have demonstrated that an iron chelator can attenuate cochlear damage from noise trauma in guinea pigs. It would appear from the published literature that iron toxicity is involved in many forms of hearing loss. It might be expected that the well-known "ringing in the ears" that many elderly men, and a few elderly women experience, will someday be linked to iron toxicology.

Iron/Aminoglycoside Complex Causes Hearing Loss

Lesniak et al. (2005) studied the mechanisms underlying the formation of reactive oxygen species by aminoglycoside antibiotics. Reactive oxygen species are suspected to be causally related to the toxic side effects of aminoglycosides to kidneys and the inner ear. The effect of iron/aminoglycoside complexes on lipid (fatty acid) metabolism was studied. Arachidonic acid, when oxidized, results in the formation of obnoxious prostaglandins. Lesniak et al. (2005) found that the iron/gentamicin complex forms a further complex with arachidonic acid, resulting in oxidation of arachidonic acid. Feldman et al.(2007) report that oral administration of 600 mg N-acetylcysteine twice daily significantly ameliorates gentamicin-induced ototoxicity in hemodialysis patients.

Superficial Siderosis of the Brain Results in Hearing Loss

Anderson et al. (1999) studied a condition known as superficial siderosis of the central nervous system. This is a late complication of cerebellar tumors. Although this condition affects only a few individuals, it sheds light on the effect of iron (in this case superficial iron on the brain detected by radiologic features). Conclusions: "Superficial siderosis is an uncommon late complication of the treatment of childhood cerebellar tumor, but it is probably underrecognized. The diagnosis should be suspected in patients who present with slowly progressive sensorineural hearing loss and ataxia many years after eradication of childhood cerebellar tumor."

Iron, the Kidneys, and Chronic Kidney Disease

The relationship between iron and the kidneys follows along two lines:

1. Iron/aminoglycoside-induced kidney damage.
2. The role of iron in chronic kidney disease.

Iron/Aminoglycoside Complex Induces Kidney Damage

This part of the story begins where the last one left off. Aminoglycosides are toxic to the kidneys, as well as to the ears. One of the side effects of aminoglycosides is kidney damage. In a review article, Ozdemir et al. (2002) reported an "Experimental study on effects of deferoxamine mesilate in ameliorating cisplatin-induced nephrotoxicity." Deferioxamine, an iron chelator, was demonstrated to ameliorate cisplatin-induced nephrotoxicity. Kudo et al. (2008) demonstrated renal tubular epithelial cell damage in iron-overloaded rats. Ekor et al. (2006) used a polyphenolic anti-oxidant extract from soybeans to ameliorate renal dysfunction induced by iron/gentamicin.

Iron Excess in Chronic Kidney Disease

In an interesting review of chronic kidney disease, Swaminathan and Shah (2008) state:

> Chronic kidney disease is a worldwide health problem that affects about 10% of the population. No major advances have been made in the treatment of this common disease, which leads to end-stage kidney disease and is associated with cardiovascular events and high economic costs. We review new approaches that are currently being explored to halt progression of kidney disease. Recent findings: Redox balance plays a significant pathogenic role in the progression of kidney disease through regulation of signaling pathways, gene expression, cell proliferation, and fibrosis.... Our emphasis here is on human studies and those agents that may have a direct or indirect link to oxidative stress and catalytic (labile) iron.

Iron in Ocular Pathology

Age-related macular degeneration (AMD) is the most recently added disease of aging that is now linked to iron excess. AMD is so common that some estimates indicate that it occurs in virtually all people over age 65 in North America. Although it has been known for many years that iron overload is associated with several forms of retinal degeneration, recent evidence suggests that iron overload may also be associated with age-related macular degeneration (Dunaief 2006, He et al. 2007, Wong et al. 2007). Dunaief was first to propose this in the 2006 Cogan Lecture.

Thalassemia: Osteoporosis and Heart Disease

Women are protected from both osteoporosis and cardiovascular disease prior to menopause. However, once a woman passes menopause, both of these conditions develop. After menopause, women begin to develop osteoporosis. Between 50 and 70 years of age, women suffer more osteoporosis than men of the same age while men have more atherosclerosis. By 70 years of age, cardiovascular disease is as prevalent among women as it is among men, and osteoporosis is as prevalent among men as among women. Perhaps observations regarding thalassemia can shed some light on this interestering relationship between osteoporosis and atherosclerosis.

Thalassemia is an inherited blood disease—associated with an inability to make enough hemoglobin. People who inherit this disease die at a very young age. Periodic blood transfusions are necessary to prolong life. However, one consequence of prolonged blood transfusions is an increase in the body burden of iron and, consequently, an increase in aging. Iron chelation therapy and phlebotomy are used to remove excess iron, with limited success. We have mentioned that thalassemic children who have been transfused have decreased bone mass due to iron's toxicity to the skeletal system (Vogiatzi et al. 2004)

Heart disease associated with iron overload is the leading cause of mortality and one of the main causes of morbidity in ß-thalassemia (Aessopos et al. 2007). The role of iron overload in thalassemia demonstrates the toxicity of iron to both the skeletal and the cardio-vascular systems, and may help to unravel the currently mysterious relationship between atherosclerosis and osteoporosis.

Iron Effects on the Pituitary Gland and Reproductive Organs

Iron Deposited in the Pituitary Gland

The pituitary gland is exceptionally sensitive to iron; as little as 1.0 micromolar of iron can completely prevent growth (Garrison, ed. 2005, p 67). The pituitary gland is a target organ in the iron overload diseases, hereditary hemochromatosis and ß-thalassemia, in which iron tends to accumulate in the anterior portion of the pituitary gland. The pituitary gland secretes gonadotrophin, which regulates functions of the sex organs. As a consequence, some people with hereditary hemochromatosis and people with ß-thalassemia develop hypogonadotrophic hypogonadism. People with thalassemia experience delayed puberty as well. A method for assessing pituitary iron overload using magnetic resonance imaging (MRI) has been developed (Argyropoulou et al. 2000; Zafar et al. 2007).

Sperm Damage Due to Iron Overload: ß-Thalassaemia

Perera et al. (2002) reported on "Sperm DNA damage in potentially fertile homozygous ß-thalassaemic patients with iron overload." The authors collected sperm from six thalassaemic patients and five age-matched controls, finding more sperm damage in thalassemics than in controls. To put this in perspective, Perera et al. state:

> Homozygous ß-thalassaemia is a hereditary haemoglobinopathy that affects >1.5 million people worldwide. Improvement of the basic management protocol of high red cell transfusion therapy has improved the longevity of the patients at least to their fourth decade. However, these patients have variable degrees of organ damage and endocrinopathies that can affect their quality of life. Hypogonadotrophic hypogonadism is the commonest

endrocrinopathy, affecting 80-90% of patients worldwide, for which homozygous ß-thalassemia major patients have disturbance of growth, sexual maturation and impaired infertility. This is largely due to iron overload.

Sperm Damage Due to Iron Overload: Animal Studies

A number of studies in rats and mice have demonstrated sperm damage by iron overload. Lucesoli and Fraga (1995) reported "oxidative damage to lipids and DNA concurrent with decrease of antioxidants in rat testes after acute iron intoxication." Lacesoli and Fraga (1999) were able to partially prevent oxidative damage to rat testes by supplementation with alpha tocopherol. Lacesoli et al. (1999) demonstrated that damage to rat testes by iron overload is dose-dependent (the more iron, the greater the damage).

Wellejus et al. (2000) demonstrated iron overload induced DNA damage to rat sperm and kidney cells in vivo and in vitro. Rajesh Kumar et al. (2002) reported on "Oxidative stress associated DNA damage in testes of mice: induction of abnormal sperms and effects on fertility." Doreswamy and Muralidhara (2005) reported, "Genotoxic consequences associated with oxidative damage in testes of mice subjected to iron intoxication." Whittaker et al. (1997) reported genetic damage in mice with iron overload.

Iron and Porphyria Cutanea Tarda (PCT)

"If I had my way, dietary iron would carry a warning label, a Commission would be appointed to study the effects of iron as a food additive, and blood tests for iron overload would become as common as a 'Pap' smear."

(Warder 1984. p xiv)

Marie Warder (1984) introduced the term, "the bronze killer," to describe her husband's manifestation of hereditary hemochromatosis. The term, "the bronze killer," has become widely used throughout the world to describe porphyria cutanea tarda (PCT). Darkening of the skin and photosensitivity are characteristic of PCT. In her book, *The Bronze Killer*, Marie Warder (1984) tells the story of her family's battle with PCT, a condition frequently associated with hereditary hemochromatosis. Even before discovery of the two major gene mutations responsible for hereditary hemochromatosis, evidence of the hereditary nature of PCT and its relationship with hemochromatosis was emerging (Fargion et al. 1996).

PCT is the most commonly recognized disorder of porphyrin metabolism. Porphyrin, made in the liver, gives rise to the porphyrin ring structure, heme, which binds iron(II). In PCT, there is a partial block of the metabolic pathway leading to heme. This causes a build up of one of the metabolites leading to prophyrin synthesis—uroporphyrin I. Clinically, PCT is characterized by photosensitive dermatitis and, biochemically, by excessive hepatic synthesis and urinary excretion of uroporphyrin I (Kushner et al. 1972). Elevated serum ferritin has been a recognized marker for PCT since 1986 (Rocchi et al. 1986).

The relationship between hemochromatosis and PCT was firmly established in 1999 (Sampietro et al. 1999). In 2001, Trombini et al. (2001) found in Italian patients that a gene mutation known as S65C results in iron accumulation when this gene occurs in heterozygous state with the C282Y and H63D gene mutations associated with hereditary hemochromatosis.

Iron and Sudden Infant Death Syndrome

Moore et al. (1994) state: "To determine the biological significance of high concentrations of non-haeme iron in the livers of infants dying from sudden infant death syndrome (SIDS), liver samples were obtained at necropsy from 66 infants who died from SIDS and 28 control infants who died before 2.5 years of age. All were full term deliveries. Liver iron concentrations decreased rapidly with age in the two groups. Liver iron concentrations the SIDS infants was 296 micrograms/g wet weight; significantly higher than the median of 105 micrograms/g in controls.... These findings show that peak incidence of SIDS occurs when mean concentrations of iron in liver tissue are higher than at any other time of life. Although a primary causal connection seems unlikely, high tissue iron concentrations may lower resistance to infection and enhance free radical formation, leading to tissue damage."

Raha-Chowdbury et al. (1996) found elevated serum ferritin and liver iron in infants dying of SIDS, and state, "Liver iron concentrations have been shown to be higher in victims of SIDS than in postmortem controls, suggesting that high levels of tissue iron may be implicated in SIDS.

Weinberg (Garrison, ed. 2005, pp 151-9) has written a review of current knowledge of the relationship between high iron stores and SIDS."

A Note of Caution to Endurance Athletes

This section is dedicated to Lance Armstrong and the LiveStrong Foundation.

Most of this book has dealt with iron toxicology as it relates to diseases of aging, and to a limited extent during infancy. However, endurance athletes may be the group most at risk for iron-excess disease as a result of taking iron supplements for exercise anemia, or engaging in blood doping. In their article, "Increased body iron stores in elite road cyclists" Deugnier et al. (2002) state:

> **Background:** One third of French elite road cyclists were found to have ferritinemia on antidoping control tests performed during the Tour de France in 1998.
>
> **Purpose:** This study was undertaken to determine whether hyperferritinemia corresponded to elevated body iron stores or not, and affirmatively, what is the mechanism, its clinical consequences, and its spontaneous course.
>
> **Methods:** 83 elite road male cyclists presenting with hyperferritinemia, defined as serum ferritin level greater than 300 microg L^{-1}, were studied with respect to consumption of iron and other drugs, serum iron tests, HFE mutation, and hepatic iron concentration.
>
> **Results:** All cyclists were asymptomatic and had normal physical and cardiac examination. Their median (range) serum ferritin, serum iron, and transferrin saturation levels were 504 microg. L^{-1} (306-1671), 20 micromol.L^{-1} (8.5-36), and 39%

(20-76), respectively. Hepatic iron was increased in 24/27 up to 187 micromol.g[-1]... Most cyclists (89%) had been supplemented with iron. The median iron supplementation was 25.5 g (range: 1.4-336) and correlated well (P = 0.002) with serum ferritin. Elevation of serum ferritin levels did not differ whether cyclists had been continuing iron supplementation or not.

Conclusion: Hyperferritinemia in elite road cyclists accounted for increased body iron stores caused by, and persisting after, cessation of excessive iron supplementation. Even when mild, iron excess may expose to long-term complications and should be removed, at least at the time when professional cyclists retire. To prevent iatrogenic iron overload, supplementation with iron must be done according to serum ferritin follow-up and not either blindly or on the basis of serum iron determination only.

REFERENCES

Aessopos A, Kati M, Farmakis D. 2007. Heart disease in thalassemia intermedia: a review of underlying pathophysiology. Hematologica. 92(5):658-65.

Anderson NE, Sheffield S, Hope JK. 1999. Superficial siderosis of the central nervous system: a late complication of cerebellar tumors. Neurology. 52(1):163-9.

Andrews NC. 1999. Disorders of iron metabolism. N Engl J Med. 341:1986-95.

Argyropoulou MI, Metafratzi Z, Kiortsis DN, Bitsis S, Tsatsoulis A, Efremidis S. 2000. T2 relaxation rate as an index of pituitary iron overload in patients with ß-thalassemia major. AJR. 175:1567-1569.

Bates DE. 2003. Aminoglycoside ototoxicity. Drugs Today (Barc). 39(4):277-85.

Blumenthal HT, Lansing AI, Wheeler PA. 1944. Calcification of the media of the human aorta and its relation to intimal arteriosclerosis, ageing, and disease. Amer J Pathol. 20:655.

Brewer GJ. 2007. Iron and copper toxicity in disease of aging, particularly atherosclerosis and Alzheimer's disease. Exp Biol Med. 232:323-35.

Chang EF, Claus CP, Vreman HJ, Wong RJ, Noble-Haeusslein LJ. 2005. Heme regulation in traumatic brain injury: relevance to adult and developing brain. J Cerebral Blood Flow & Metab. 25:1401-17.

Chau LY. 2000. Iron and atherosclerosis. Proc Natl Sci Repub China

B. 24(4):151-5.

Chen Y, Wang J, Huang W. 1999. [Desferrioxamine protects against getamicin ototoxicity]. Zhonghua Er Bi Yan Hou Ke Za Zhi. 34(3):154-6. [In Chinese]

Chua-anusorn W, Webb J, Macey DJ, de la Motte, Hall P, St Pierre TG. 1999. The effect of prolonged iron loading on the chemical form of iron oxide deposits in rat liver and spleen. Biochim Biophys Acta. 1454(2):191-200.

Conlon BJ, Perry BP, Smith DW. 1998. Attenuation of neomycin ototoxicity by iron chelation. Laryngoscope. 108(2):284-7.

Deugnier Y, Loréal O, Carré F, Duvallet A, Zoulin F, Vinel JP, Paris JC, Blaison D, Moirand R, Turlin B, Gandon Y, David V, Mégret A, Guinot M. 2002. Increased body iron stores in elite road cyclists. Med Sci Sports Exerc. 34(5):876-80.

Doreswami K, Muralidhara. 2005. Genotoxic consequences associated with oxidative damage in testis of mice subjected to iron intoxication. Toxicology. 206(1):169-78.

Dunaief JL. 2006. Iron induced oxidative damage as a potential factor in age-related macular degeneration: the Cogan Lecture. Invest Ophthalmology 112:1062-5.

Ekor M, Farombi EO, Emerole GO. 2006. Modulation of hentamicin-induced renal dysfunction and injury by phenolic extract of soybean (Glycine Max). Fundam Clin Pharmacol. 20(3):263-71.

Erdemoglu AK, Ozbakir S. 2002. Serum ferritin levels and early prognosis of stroke. Eur J Neurol. 9(6):633-7.

Facchini FS. 2002. *The Iron Factor of Aging. Why Do Americans Age Faster?* Tucson: Fenestra Books.

Fargion S, Fracanzani AL, Romano R, Cappellini MD, Faré M, Mattioli M, Piperano A, Ronchi G, Fiorelli G. 1996. Genetic hemochromatosis in Italian patients with porphyria cutanea tarda: possible explanation for iron overload. Hepatol. 24(5):564-9.

Feldman L, Efrati S, Eviatar E, Abramsohn R, Yarovow I, Gersch E, Averbukh Z, Weissgarten J. 2007. Gentamicin-induced ototoxicity in hemodialysis patients is ameliorated by N-acetylcysteine. Kidney Int. 72(3):359-63.

Fleming DJ, Tucker KL, Jacques PR, Dallal GE, Wilson PWF, Wood RJ. 2002. Dietary factors associated with the risk of high iron stores in the elderly Framingham Heart Study cohort. Am J Clin Nutr. 76:1375-84.

Garrison C, ed. 2001. *Iron Disorders Institute. Guide to Hemochroma-*

tosis. Nashville: Cumberland House.

———— 2003. *Iron Disorders Institute. Guide to Hemochromatosis.* Nashville: Cumberland House.

———— 2005. *Exposing the Hidden Dangers of Iron.* By Weinberg ED. Nashville: Cumberland House.

Guggenbuhl P, Deugnier Y, Boisdet JF, Rolland Y, Perdriger A, Pawlotsky Y, Chalds G. 2005. Bone mineral densiry in men with genetic hemochromatosis and HFE gene mutation. Osteoporos Int. 16(12):1809-14.

He X, Hahn P, Iacovelli J, Wong R, King C, Bhisitkul R, Massaro-Giordano M, Dunaief JL. 2007. Progress in Retinal and Eye Research. 26: 649-73.

Herbert V. 1994. Iron worsens high-cholesterol-related coronary artery disease. Am J Clin Nutr. 60:299-302.

Hua Y, Keep RF, Hoff, JT, Xi G. 2007. Brain injury after intracerebral hemorrhage. The role of thrombin and iron. Stroke. 38[part 2]:759-62.

Jiang R, Manson JAE, Meigs JB, Ma Jing, Rifai N, Hu FB. 2004. Body iron stores in relation to risk of type 2 diabetes in apparently healthy women. JAMA. 291(6):711-17.

Kudo H, Suzuki S, Watanabe A, Kikuchi H, Sassa S, Sakamoto S. 2008. Effects of iron overload on renal and hepatic siderosis and the femur in male rats. Toxicology. [Epub ahead of print]

Kushner JP, Lee GR, Macht S. 1972. The role of iron in pathogenesis of porphyria cutanea tarda. J Clin Invest. 51(12):3044-51.

Lauffer RB. 1993. *Iron and Your Heart.* New York: St. Martin's Press.

Lautermann J, Dehne N, Schacht J, Jahnke K. 2004. [Aminoglycoside- and cisplatin-ototoxicity: from basic science to clinics]. Laryngorhinootologie. 83(5):317-23. [In German]

Lesniak W, Pecoraro VL, Schacht J. 2005. Ternary complexes of gentamicin with iron and lipid catalyzed formation of reactive oxygen species. Chem Res Toxicol. 18(2):357-64.

Lucesoli F, Fraga CG. 1995. Oxidative damage to lipids and DNA concurrent with decrease antioxidants in rat testes after acute iron intoxication. Arch Biochem Biophys. 31(6):5678-71.

———— 1999. Oxidative stress in testes of rats subjected to iron intoxication and alpha-tocopherol supplementation. Toxicology. 132(2):179-86.

Lucesoli G, Caligiuri M, Roberti MF, Perazzo JC, Frage CG. 1999. Dose-dependent increase of oxidative damage in the testes of rats subjected to acute iron overload. 372(1):37-43.

Meyers DG. 1996. The iron hypothesis—does iron cause atherosclerosis? Clin Cardiol. 19(12):925-9.

Millan, M, Sobrino T, Caswtellanos M, Nombela F, Arenillas JF, Riva E, Cristobo I, Garcìa MM, Vivancos J, Serena J, Morro MA, Castillo J, Dávalos A. 2007. Increased body iron stores are associated with poor outcome after thrombolytic treatment in acute stroke. Stroke. 38:90-5.

Moore CA, Raha-Chowdhury R, Fagan DG, Worwood M. 1994. Liver iron concentrations in sudden infant death syndrome. 70($):295-8.

Ozdemir E, Dokucu AI, Uzunlar AK, Ece A, Yaldiz AK, Ece A, Yaldiz M, Oztürk H. 2002. Experimental study on effects of deferoxamine mesilate in emeliorating cisplatin-induced nephrotoxicity. Int Urol Nephrol. 33(1):127-31.

Papanastasiou DA, Vayenas DV, Vassilopoulos A, Repanti A. 2000. Concentration of iron and distribution of iron and transferrin after experimental iron overload in rat tissues in vivo: study of the liver, the spleen, the nervous system, and other organs. Pathol Res Pract. 196(1):47-54.

Pereira MC, Pereira ML, Sousa JP. 1999. Histological effects of iron accumulation on mice liver and spleen after administration of a metallic solution. Biomaterials. 20(22):2193-8.

Perera D, Pizzey A, Campbell A, Katz M, Porter J, Petrou M, Irvine DS, Chatterjee R. 2002. Sperm DNA damage in potentially fertile homozygous ß-thalassaemia patients with iron overload. Human Reproduction. 17(7):1820-5.

Raha-Chowhury R, Moore CA, Bradley D, Henley R, Worwood M. 1996. Blood ferritin concentrations in newborns and the sudden infant death syndrome. J Clin Pathol. 49:168-70.

Rajesh Kumar T, Doreswamy K, Shrilatha B, Muralidhra. 2002. Oxidative stress associated DNA damage in testis of mice: induction of abnormal sperms and effects on fertility. Mutat Res. 513(1,2):103-11.

Rocchi E, Gibertini P, Cassanelli M, Pietrangelo A, Borghi A, Ventura E. 1986. Serum ferritin in the assessment of liver iron overload and iron removal therapy in porphyria cutanea tarda. Lab Clin Med. 107(1):36-42.

Sampietro M, Fiorelli G, Fargion S. 1999. Iron overload in porphyria cutanea tarda. Haematologica. 84:248-53.

Song BB, Anderson DJ, Schacht J. 1997. Protection from gentamicin ototoxicity by iron chelators in guinea pig *in vivo*. J Pharmacol Exp Therap. 282:369-77.

Song BB, Sha SH, Schacht J. 1998. Iron chelators protect from aminoglycoside-induced cochleo- and vestibulo-toxicity. Free Radic Biol Med. 25(2):189-95.

Sullivan JL. 1981. Iron and the sex differences in heart disease risk. Lancet. 1(8233):1293-4.

———— 1992. Stored iron as a risk factor for ischemic heart disease. In: Lauffer RB, ed. *Iron and Human Disease.* Boca Raton, Ann Arbor, London, Tokyo: CRC Press.

Swaminathan S, Shah SV. 2008. Novel approaches targeted toward oxidative stress for the treatment of chronic kidney disease. Curr Opin Nephrol Hypertens. 17(2):143-8.

Terada LS, Willingham IR, Repine JE. 1992. Iron and stroke. In: *Iron and Human Disease.* Boca Raton, Ann Arbor, London, Tokyo: CRC Press, p 313-332.

Trobini P, Mauri V, Salvioni A, Corengia C, Arosio C, Piperno A. 2001. S65C frequency in Italian patients with hemochromatosis, porphyria cutanea tarda and viral hepatitis with iron overload. Hematologica. 86:316-7.

van der A DL, Grobbee DE, Roest M, Mars JJ, Voorbij HA, van der Schouw YT. 2005. Serum ferritin is a risk factor for stroke in postmenopausal. 36(8):1637-41.

Vayanes DV, Repanti M, Vassilopoulor A, Papenstasiou DA. 1998. Influence of iron overload on magnesium, zinc, and copper concentration in rat tissues in vivo. Study of liver, spleen, and brain. Int J Clin Lab Res. 28(3):183-6.

Vogiatzi MG, Autio KA, Schneider R, Giardina PJ. 2004. Low bone mass in prepubertal children with Thalassemia major: insights into the pathogenesis of low bone mass in Thalassemia. J Ped Endocrinol & Metab. 17:1415-21.

Warder, M. 1984. *The Bronze Killer. Hemochromatosis: The No. 1 Genetic Disorder.* Delta, BC, Canada: Imperani Publishers.

Weinberg ED. 2001. Elevated iron, antibiotics and hearing loss. Iron Disorders Institute. 2nd Quarter 2001, p 9.

———— 2006. Iron loading: a risk factor for osteoporosis. BioMetals. 19:633-35.

Wellejus A, Poulsen HD, Loft S. 2000. Iron-induced oxidative DNA damage in rat sperm cells in vivo and in vitro. Free Radic Res. 32(1):75-83.

Whittaker P, Dunkel VC, Bucci TJ, Kusewitt DF, Thurman JD, Warbritton A, Wolff GL. 1997. Genome-linked toxic responses to dietary iron overload. Toxicol Pathol. 25(6):556-64.

Whittaker P, Hines FA, Robl MG, Dunkel VC. 1996. Histopathological evaluation of liver, pancreas, spleen, and heart from iron-overloaded Sprague-Dawley rats. Toxicol Path. 24(5):558-63.

Witte DL, Crosby WH, Edwards CO, Fairbanks VF, Mitros FA. 1996. Practice guideline development task force of the College of American Pathologists: hereditary hemochromatosis. Clin Chim Acta. 245:139-200.

Wong RW, Richa DC, Hahn P, Green WR, Dunaief JL. 2007. Iron toxicity as a potential factor in AMD. Retina. 27:997-1003.

Yamasoba T, Schacht J, Shoji F, Miller JM. 1999. Attenuation of chochlear damage from nois trauma by an iron chelator, a free radical scavenger and glial cell-line-derived neutrotrophic factor in vivo. Brain Res. 815(2):317-25.

You S-A, Archacki SR. Angheloiu G, Moravee CS,Rao S, Kinter M, Topol, EJ, Wang Q. 2003. Proteomic approach to coronary atherosclerosis shows ferritin light chain as a significant marker: evidence consistent with the iron hypothesis in atherosclerosis. Physiol Genomics. 13:25-30.

Zacharski LR, Ornstein DL, Woloshin S, Schwartz LM. 2000. Association of age, sex, and race with body iron stores in adults: analysis of NHANES III data. Am Heart J. 140(1):98-104.

Zafar AM, Zuberi L, Khan AH, Ahsan H. 2007. Utility of MRI in assessment of pituitary iron overload. Pak Med Assoc. 57(9):475-7.

Chapter 8

The Best Defense

Introduction

The fundamental reason for iron's toxicity resides in the ability of iron to redox cycle with oxygen. This can occur when body iron stores are excessive. Maintaining low but adequate body iron is the goal. A low-iron, antioxidant-rich diet is the best defense against iron toxicity.

A macrobiotic diet, based on brown rice and other whole grains supplemented with vegetables, legumes, seeds, and nuts, is ideal from the standpoint of iron nutrition. Several macrobiotic cookbooks are available, including *Basic Macrobiotic Cooking* by Julia Ferré, *Self-Healing Cookbook* by Kristina Turner, and *Complete Guide to Macrobiotic Cooking* by Aveline Kushi. A good introduction to macrobiotic theory and practice is *Pocket Guide to Macrobiotics* by Carl Ferré.

In addition, there are a number of books with recipes, food tables, and advice on how to lower the iron content of your diet. Two of these are: *The Hemochromatosis Cookbook: Recipes and Menus for Reducing the Iron in Your Diet* by C. Garrison and A. Rasswater; and *Iron Balance: The New "Iron-Lite" Health Plan that Restores Your Inner Vitality* by R. B. Lauffer, PhD.

In this section, we will discuss the difference between organic and inorganic iron, followed by a discussion of the roles of various nutrients and procedures for maintaining low but adequate iron stores, i.e., maintaining iron balance.

1. **Iron chelating agents in food**. We will begin with the important iron-chelating, antioxidant nutrients: phytate, lactoferrin, and ovotransferrin.
2. **Other antioxidants in food**. The importance of antioxidants other than iron chelating agents: polyphenols, vitamin E, ß-carotene, and vitamin C.
3. **De-ironing**: Blood donation, aspirin, and chelation therapy.
4. **Antioxidant enzymes**: superoxide dismutase (SOD), catalase, and glutathione peroxidase.
5. **Sulfur-containing antioxidants**: Cysteine, N-acetyl cysteine, and glutathione.

The Chemical Nature of Dietary Iron

One major reason for the wide spread occurrence of iron deposition diseases in North America resides in the nature of the iron that is added to food. Prior to 1941, when the addition of iron to food was initiated, all dietary iron was chelated iron—iron bound to organic molecules. We refer to this binding of iron in an organic matrix as a chelate (claw) because the organic molecule binds the iron in claw-like fashion. In 1941, when the decision was made to add iron to milled grains, virtually nothing was known regarding iron's potential for toxicity. The argument at the time was that a certain amount of iron had been removed from grains during milling, and it was necessary to add the iron back. In fact, it was decided to add even more iron than was taken out, just to be safe.

Those who initiated the practice of adding iron to food were ignorant of the fact that iron might be toxic, or that inorganic iron would prove to be more toxic than organic iron. At the time, there was virtually no information regarding iron toxicity. However, it was well-known that phytate-bound (organic) iron is less well absorbed than inorganic iron. And, in fact, that is one of the major reasons for choosing inorganic iron as a food additive. At that time, the entire nation was taken up in the "Popeye Syndrome"—the more iron the better.

Iron in Unfortified Foods is Chelated

Iron in milk (although there is not much) is chelated by lactoferrin. Iron in egg white is chelated to ovotransferrin (ovalbumin). Iron in plants is chelated to phytate, or to one of the many plant siderophores (sidero = iron; phore refers to binding).

Heme iron

In red meat, fish, pork, chicken, and other animals, the iron is largely bound to heme or myoglobin. We have previously discussed heme iron and have observed that heme iron is more readily absorbed than is plant-derived iron. Unabsorbed heme iron may have adverse effects resulting in intestinal inflammation and colon cancer.

Organic Iron

Organic iron refers to all iron that occurs in natural food. Heme iron, phytate iron, lactoferrin iron, transferrin iron, ovotransferrin iron, siderophore iron, and all other iron contained in natural food is chelated to an organic molecule and is organic iron. There may be small amounts of iron in natural food that is not tightly chelated. This iron is ligand-bound to small organic molecules. Ligand-bound iron is not as tightly bound as is chelated iron.

Inorganic iron

Inorganic iron is most of the iron that is added to food. This book contains a list of eleven inorganic forms of iron that are FDA-approved for adding to food. These inorganic forms of iron are more readily absorbed than is organic iron. In fact, if inorganic iron is taken with vitamin C, the percent of iron absorbed is even greater than the 30 or 40% absorption estimated for heme iron. Vitamin C-iron is one of several forms of iron approved by the FDA for use as a supplement.

There are 9 ligand-bound forms of iron approved by the FDA for use in food, or as supplements. Because every ligand-form of iron results in different absorption, the FDA has opened Pandora's box, and North Americans are inundated with forms, and amounts, of iron that no other humans had previously been exposed to. The inorganic iron that is added to food also becomes ligand-bound; unfortunately, ligand binding does not prevent iron from redox cycling. In fact, as in the case of iron-ascorbate, ligand binding may promote redox cycling.

This leads to the inevitable conclusion: **The decision to add iron to food is the greatest mistake in the entire history of human nutrition; the decision to use *inorganic iron* is the second.**

With the exception of heme iron, all natural dietary sources of iron protect us from over-absorption of iron. The inorganic forms of iron that are added to food are not so protected. Inorganic iron currently constitutes around ½ of all dietary iron in North America. Evolution has provided no protection against inorganic iron, which results in continually increasing the body iron burden during the aging process in North America (Zacharaski et al. 2000, Fleming et al. 2002).

Dietary Antioxidants that Prevent Iron Overabsorption

Lactoferrin (and transferrin/ovotransferrin), phytate, and plant siderophores are antioxidants that exert their antioxidant effects in the intestinal tract. By binding iron, these antioxidants prevent iron overabsorption and prevent iron from redox cycling in the intestinal tract. Lactoferrin and phytate have been demonstrated to have anticancer properties, in particular in the prevention of colon cancer.

Dietary Lactoferrin, Ovotransferrin, and Phytate

Although it was believed in the 1940s that increased iron absorption from food would be advantageous, the vastly documented research in iron toxicology, which has developed at a dramatic rate since the 1980s, indicates that may not have been a good idea. Perhaps Nature had a better idea when She made certain that iron in all natural foods is chelated, preventing iron overabsorption. Not only does natural, organic iron prevent iron overabsorption, natural sources of iron (with the exception of heme iron) prevent iron from redox cycling in the colon and, thereby, help prevent inflammation and cancer in the lower digestive tract, colon, and rectum.

Among the most important iron-chelating substances are phytate, lactoferrin, and ovotransferrin. These are natural iron overabsorption-preventing substances and are crucial to maintaining appropriate iron homeostasis.

- **Lactoferrin** is the major iron-binding component of milk. All iron in milk is in iron-lactoferrin-chelate.
- **Ovotransferrin** is the iron-binding component of eggs. All dietary iron from egg white is iron-ovotransferrin-chelate.
- **Phytate** is the primary iron-binding component in foods of plant origin.

Lactoferrin: Lactoferrin has well-documented bacteriostatic, antiviral, anti-aging, and anti-cancer properties. It is possible that future investigations will find similar properties for transferrin and ovotransferrin. However, transferrin and ovotransferrin have not been as thoroughly studied. This mini-review will concentrate on lactoferrin. Ward et al. (2005) stated: "Lactoferrin (LF) is a member of the transferrin family that is expressed and secreted by glandular epithelial cells and is found in the secondary granules of neutrophils. Originally viewed as an iron-binding protein in milk, with bacteriostatic properties, it is becoming increasingly evident that LF is a multifunctional protein to which several physiological roles have been attributed. These include regulation of iron homeostasis, host defense against a broad range of microbial infections, anti-inflammatory activity, regulation of cellular growth, and differentiation and protection against cancer development and metastasis."

Weinberg (2007) stated: "Recombinant bovine and human lactoferrin is now available for development into nutraceutical/preservative/pharmaceutical products. Among conditions for which the products are being investigated are: angiogenesis; bone remodeling; food preservation; infection in animals, humans, plants; neoplasia in animals, humans; inflammation in intestine, joints; wound healing; as well as enhancement of antimicrobial and antineoplastic drugs, and prevention of iron induced oxidation of milk formula."

Some of the properties of lactoferrin, such as stimulation of immune system function, anti-cancer, anti-viral, and anti-bacterial properties are indicated by the following:

- "Milk and dairy products in cancer prevention: focus on bovine lactoferrin." (Tsuda et al. 2000)
- "Cancer prevention by bovine lactoferrin and underlying mechanisms—a review of experimental and clinical studies." (Tsuda et al. 2002)
- "Orally administered lactoferrin restores humoral immune response in immunocompromised mice." (Artym et al. 2003)
- "Oral lactoferrin inhibits growth of established tumors and potentiates conventional chemotherapy." (Varadhachary et al. 2004)
- "Bovine lactoferrin inhibits tumor-induced angiogenesis." (Shimamura et al. 2004)
- "Lactoferrin inhibits human papillomavirus binding and uptake in vitro." (Drobni et al. 2004)
- "Bovine lactoferrin: benefits and mechanism of action against infections." (Yamauchi et al. 2006).
- "Oral lactoferrin results in T cell-dependent tumor inhibition of head and neck squamous cell carcinoma in vivo." (Wolf et al. 2007)
- "Anti-papillomavirus activity of human and bovine lactoferrin." (Mistry et al. 2007)

Fecal lactoferrin and hemoglobin may be useful markers for colorectal disease (Hirata et al. 2007).

Conclusions: Lactoferrin is an essential component of an infant's diet and has beneficial effects beyond those of iron binding.

Lactoferrin's antibacterial, antiviral, and anticancer effects are well documented. Based on lactoferrin essentiality in an infant diet, lactoferrin is classified as an essential nutrient ("vitamin") during infancy and an important accessory food factor for adults.

Phytate: Phytate is *myo*-insotol hexaphosphate. *Myo*-insotol is a simple six-carbon sugar that was initially referred to as an accessory food factor. *Myo*-inositol is important in the formation of the lipid membranes surrounding nerves. Although *myo*-inositol is biosynthesized, infants may not be able to make it in sufficient amounts, so it is added to infant formula to promote normal brain development. *Myo*-inositol has six hydroxy groups that can be phosphorylated, resulting in several inositol phosphates. Inositol diphosphate and inositol triphosphate have important roles in cellular signaling and brain function. However, of the six possible inositol phosphates, *myo*-inositol hexaphosphate is the only inositol phosphate that can completely suppress redox cycling in *in vitro* cell studies (Hawkins et al. 1993). *Myo*-inositol hexaphosphate is also known as phytic acid, phytate, or IP_6. Tsuno Foods & Rice Co, Wakayama, Japan sells a rice bran extract high in IP_6 (Sardi 1999).

Phytate is an abundant plant constituent, comprising 1-5% by weight of edible legumes, cereals, oil seeds, pollens, and nuts. In seeds, phytate comprises more than 70% of the kernel phosphorous (Zhou and Erdman 1995). Originally believed to be the storage form of phosphorous in seeds (Hawkins et al. 1993), phytate is now also known to preserve seeds by binding iron, thereby preventing oxidative damage due to iron redox cycling (Graff et al. 1987, Graff and Eaton 1990, Rimbach and Pallauf 1998). Dietary phytate protects the colon from lipid peroxidation in pigs on a high iron diet (Porres et al. 1999); protects rats from carcinogen-induced colon cancer (Nelson et al. 1989, Owen et al. 1998); and ameliorates pulmonary inflammation induced by asbestos in a rat model (Kamp et al. 1995). Because phytate may play a role in colon cancer prevention, a method for determining fecal phytate as a potential marker of risk for colon cancer has been developed (Owen et al. 1996).

Other Dietary Antioxidants

Vitamin E, ß-carotene, vitamin C, and polyphenols are the best-known plant-derived antioxidants. Vitamin E, ß-carotene, and vitamin C are vitamins, whereas polyphenols are not considered to be vitamins—at least not in North America, although bioflavonoids are referred to as vitamin P in Europe. Following are brief comments on the major groups of antioxidants.

Vitamin E

Vitamin E is also known as tocopherol. There are several tocopherols, such as alpha-tocopherol, gamma-tocopherol, and others, all of which act as antioxidants. Tocopherols are lipids (fats), and are found in the membrane of every healthy cell where they squeeze between cholesterol and polyunsaturated fatty acids, phospholipids, and other components of the lipid bilayer. The tocopherols accept electrons that are generated within the lipid bilayer.

The tocopherols operate in harmony with vitamin C, which is found in the cytoplasm of the cell because it is water soluble. Vitamin E regenerates by donating electrons to vitamin C at the water/lipid interface. Vitamin C disperses the electron into the cytoplasmic matrix. This process protects the cell membrane (lipid bilayer) from sustaining damage due to the release of the electrons within the membrane.

Many studies have shown beneficial effects of vitamin E in heart disease, cancer, and other diseases. Good sources of vitamin E are nuts, whole grains, and wheat germ oil.

Polyphenols

The polyphenols have enjoyed a great deal of publicity in recent years due to their abundance in tea and red wine, so the reader is probably aware that the polyphenols are antioxidants. A literature search on polyphenols via PubMed yielded over 2000 scientific publications, most of them published since 2000!

There are hundreds, perhaps thousands, of polyphenols. D'Archivio et al (2007) presents information on occurrence and classification of polyphenols: "Polyphenols are the most abundant antioxidants in our diet and are widespresd constituents of fruits, vegetables, cereals, olives, dry legumes, chocolate, and beverages, such as tea, coffee and wine....The main groups of polyphenols are: flavonoids, phenolic acids, phenolic alcohols, stilbenes, and lignans."

In addition to being antioxidants, the polyphenols have important anti-inflammatory activity (Santangelo et al. 2007). Part of the antioxidant properties of polyphenols is due to iron binding; however, polyphenols have additional antioxidant properties that are only now being explored. Polyphenols play an important, but so far unexplained, role on the process of apoptosis. Apoptosis is a form of cell death that plays an important role in normal embryonic development. In adults, apoptosis maintains tissue homeostasis. (Giovannini et al. 2007).

Quercetin

Quercitin is one of the polyphenols of greatest interest. As stated above, there are six chemical classes of polyphenols. Flavonoids are one of these classes. The flavonoids are themselves divided into six subclasses. The flavonols are one of these subclasses—quercetin is one of many flavonols. The flavonols represent the most ubiquitous flavonoids in foods, with quercetin as the most representative compound. Main sources of flavonols are onions, apple (especially the peel), kale, leeks, broccoli, and blueberries.

Quercetin is an important nutrient that has been demonstrated to strengthen the immune system, lower blood pressure, reduce heart attacks, protect from cancer, and has many other beneficial effects. Quercetin has antioxidant properties that include iron-binding but go beyond that. In fact, quercetin (and presumably other flavanols) are the only known naturally occurring substances that can prevent formation of the hydroxyl radical. The mechanisms by which quercetin exerts its effects are becoming known and will be recorded in an upcoming book, *Nutrition Discoveries and Mistakes of the 20th Century.*

Quercetin is available commercially at a Web site hosted by Lance Armstrong: *http://www.healthyenergy.com.*

Vitamin C

Vitamin C has both antioxidant and prooxidant properties and must be considered separately from other nutritional antioxidants. By reducing iron(III) to iron(II), vitamin C increases iron absorption. Vitamin C may also redox cycle with iron in the intestinal tract and generate oxygen radicals. Consuming too much vitamin C with an iron-rich diet may be dangerous. Vitamin C is also known as ascorbic acid, which is the term I will use here.

Because ascorbic acid synthesized in a laboratory is identical in chemical composition to ascorbic acid that occurs in plants, it has been argued that taking laboratory-synthesized ascorbic acid is just as good as taking natural ascorbic acid. That reasoning is not altogether right in view of current knowledge of iron toxicology. All natural sources of ascorbic acid contain polyphenols which, by chelating iron, prevent the obnoxious effects of ascorbic acid-iron interactions. Albert Szent-Györgyi, who discovered ascorbic acid, also discovered a group of nutrients that could prevent fragility of the microvasculature of the skin and, therefore, help prevent bruising. Szent-Györgyi designated the citrus bioflavonoids, "vitamin P." The citrus bioflavonoids never did become recognized as vitamins in the United States, but they are in the European Community. The polyphenols are now proven to be essential dietary components with anti-aging, vitamin-like properties.

The role of ascorbic acid in iron toxicology argues against taking laboratory-synthesized ascorbic acid, especially if it is combined with iron.

De-Ironing

Because there is no physiological mechanism for excreting iron, removal of iron from people with high iron burden can be accomplished only by removing blood, or administering a drug that can bring about iron excretion. Blood contains around 0.5 mg iron/ml.

Aspirin causes microbleeding in the intestine and can, therefore, remove a fair amount of iron. Regular blood donation can remove even more.

Chelating agents can be used, by prescription. People with hereditary hemochromatosis and people such as thalassemics who need regular blood transfusions are treated by chelation therapy. The powerful iron chelator, deferrioxamine, has been available for many years. Ferrioxamine is one of the plant siderophores—the first one discovered. When iron is removed from ferrioxamine, it is referred to as deferrioxamine. Deferrioxamine is administered by injection, which is not always suitable. Deferasirox is a newer version of deferrioxamine that can be taken orally. Deferasirox is manufactured by Novartis Pharmaceuticals and is marketed under the trade name, Exjade.

What blood levels of iron should accompany the process of de-ironing? According to Weinberg (Garrison, ed. 2005, p 217), "De-ironing is complete when ferritin reaches 25 ng/ml on one occasion (while pretreatment hemoglobin remains at 12.5 g/dL or greater). Therefore, to avoid anemia-related symptoms such as restless legs syndrome, serum ferritin should remain in a range of 25-75 ng/mL with an accompanying transferrin saturation percentage <40 percent."

Antioxidant Enzymes

Antioxidant enzymes are made within the body. These include superoxide dismutase, catalase, and glutathione peroxidase. In general, we have no control over the synthesis of these enzymes, with the exception of glutathione peroxidase, which may be increased by eating selenium-rich foods.

Glutathione Peroxidase/Selenium

Hydrogen peroxide is continually being generated within cells and could cause oxidative damage if not removed. Glutathione peroxidase is a selenium-containing enzyme that removes hydrogen peroxide. Selenium has antioxidant properties due to its incorporation into glutathione peroxidase, and is added to many nutritional supplements. The unique smell of garlic is due to selenium; thus, garlic is a rich source of selenium, as are many other plants.

Superoxide Dismutase (SOD)

Superoxide dismutase (SOD) is an enzyme that removes the superoxide radical—an oxygen radical that could be exceptionally damaging to biomolecules. SOD was discovered in 1969 by McCord and Fridovich (1969). It was soon demonstrated that the more SOD an animal has, the longer the lifespan. This suggested that if we could increase our SOD, we could increase our longevity. SOD found its way into health food stores where it was promoted as the "Eternity Enzyme." Unfortunately, superoxide dismutase is destroyed in the intestinal tract, as most proteins are, and does not bring about the desired increase. Still, someone made a fortune selling it!

Sulfur-containing Antioxidants:

Glutathione is a tripeptide, gamma-glutamylcysteinylglycine. The reason for giving this somewhat tedious name is to indicate that glutathione is a tripeptide that contains cysteine. Cysteine is one of two sulfur-containing amino acids. Iron and sulfur are like yang and yin—a very happy couple. The affinity these two elements have for each is incredible. However, many of the toxic metals also have a high affinity for sulfur. The competition between iron and mercury, lead, or cadmium for cysteinyl sulfur is one of the foundations of metal toxicology in general, which is the topic of the next book in this series.

Final Remarks

This book is first in a series of three. Although we have dealt extensively with iron toxicology in this book, we have presented very little information regarding the biochemistry of iron. Book II, *En-*

vironmental Toxicology of Metals, will examine the biochemistry of iron, and the toxicology of mercury, lead, cadmium, manganese, thallium, silver, arsenic, and other toxic metals in the environment. Book III will consider *Nutrition Advances and Mistakes of the Twentieth Century*.

I hope you have enjoyed reading this book, and that it will help you find better health.

REFERENCES

Artym J, Zimecki M, Paprocka M, Kruzel ML. 2003. Orally administered lactoferrin restores humoral immune response in immunocompromised mice. Immunol Lett. 89(1):9-15.

D'Archivio MD, Filesi C, Di Benedetto R, Gargiulo R. 2007. Polyphenols, dietary sources and bioavailability. Ann Ist Super Sanita. 43(4):348-61.

Drobni P, Näslund J, Evander M. 2004. Antiviral Res. Lactoferrin inhibits human papillomavirus binding and uptake in vitro. Antiviral Res. 64(1):63-8.

Ferré, C. 1997. *Pocket Guide to Macrobiotics*. Berkeley, CA: Crossing Press.

Ferré, J. 2007. *Basic Macrobiotic Cooking: Twentieth Anniversary Edition*. Chico, CA: George Ohsawa Macrobiotic Foundation.

Fleming DJ, Tucker KL, Jacques PR, Dallal GE, Wilson PWF, Wood RJ. 2002. Dietary factors associated with the risk of high iron stores in the elderly Framingham Heart Study cohort. Am J Clin Nutr. 76:1375-84.

Garrison C, ed. 2005. *Exposing the Hidden Dangers of Iron*. By Weinberg ED. Nashville, TN: Cumberland House.

Garrison C, Rasswater A. 2008. *The Hemochromatosis Cookbook: Recipes and Menus for Reducing the Iron in Your Diet*.

Giovannini C, Scazzocchio B, Vari R, Santangelo C, D'Achivio M, Masella R. 2007. Apoptosis in cancer and atherosclerosis: polyphenol activities. Ann Ist Super Sanita, 43(4):406-16.

Graf E, Eaton JW. 1990. Antioxidant functions of phytic acid. Free Radic Biol Med. 8(1):61-9.

Graf E, Empsos KL. 1987. Phytic acid: a natural antioxidant. JBC. 262(24):11647-50.

Hawkins PT, Poyner DR, Jackson TR, Letcher AJ, Lander DA, Irvine RF. 1993. Inhibition of iron-catalysed hydroxyl radical formation by inositol polyphosphates: a possible physiological function for *myo*-inositol hexakisphosphate. Biochem J. 294:929-34.

Hirata I, Hoshimoto M, Saito O, Kayazawa M, Nishikawa T, Murano M, Toshina K, Wang FY, Matsuse R. 2007. Usefulness of fecal lactoferrin and hemoglobin in diagnosis of colorectal disease. World J Gastroenterol. 13(10):1569-74.

Kamp DW, Israbian VA, Yeidandi AV, Panos RJ, Graceffa P, Weitzman SA. 1995. Phytic acid, an iron chelator, attenuates pulmonary inflammation and fibrosis in rats after intratracheal instillation of asbestos. Toxicol Pathol. 23(6):689-95.

Kushi, A. 1985. *Complete Guide to Macrobiotic Cooking*. New York: Warner Books.

Lauffer RB. 1991. *Iron Balance. The New "Iron-Lite" Health Plan that Restores Your Inner Vitality*. New York: St Martin's Press.

McCord JM, Fridovich I. 1969. Superoxide dismutase: an enzymic function for erythroprein (hemocuprein). J Biol Chem. 244:6049.

Mistry N, Drobini P, Näslund J, Sunkari VG, Jenssen H, Evander M. 2007. Anti-papillomavirus activity of human and bovine lactoferrin. Antiviral Res. 75(3):258-65.

Nelson RL, Yoo SJ, Tanure JC, Andrianopoulos G, Misumi A. 1989. Anticancer Res. 9(6):1477-82.

Owen RW, Spiegelhalder B, Bartsch H. 1998. Phytate, reactive oxygen species and colorectal cancer. Eur J Cancer Prev. 7 Suppl 2:S41-54.

Owen RW, Weisgerber UM, Spiegelhalder B, Bartsch H. 1996. Faecal phytic acid and its relation other putative markers of risk of colorectal cancer. Gut. 38:591-7.

Porres JM, Stahl CC, Cheng WH, Fu Y, Roneker KR, Pond WG, Lei XG. 1999. Dietary intrinsic phytate protects colon from lipid peroxidation in pigs with a moderately high dietary iron intake. Proc Soc Exp Biol Med. 221(1):80-6.

Rimbach G, Pallauf J. 1998. Phytic acid inhibits free radical formation in vitro but does not affect liver oxidant or antioxidant status in growing rats. J Nutr. 128(11):1950-5.

Santangelo C, Vari R, Seazzocchio B, De Benedetto R, Filesi C, Masella R. 2007. Polyphenols, intracellular signaling and inflammation. Ann Ist Super Sanita. 43(4):394-405.

Sardi B. 1999. *The Iron Time Bomb*. San Dimas, CA: Bill Sardi.

Shimamura M, Yamamoto Y, Ashino H, Oikawa T, Hazato T, Tsuda H, Iigo M. 2004. Bovine lactoferrin inhibits tumor-induced angiogenesis. Int

J Cancer. 111(1):111-6.

Tsuda H, Sekine K, Ushida Y, Kuhara T, Takasuka N, Iigo M, Han BS, Moore MA. Milk and dairy products in cancer prevention: focus on bovine lactoferrin. 2000. Mutat Res. 462(2-3):227-33.

Tsuda H, Sekine K, Fujita K, Ligo M. 2002. Cancer prevention by bovine lactoferrin and underlying mechanisms – a review of experimental and clinical studies. Biochem Cell Biol. 80(1):131-6.

Turner, K. 1987. *Self-Healing Cookbook.* Vashon Island, WA: Earthtones Press.

Varadhachary A, Wolf JS, Petrak K, O'Malley BW Jr, Spadaro M, Curcio C, Forni G, Pericle F.2004. Oral lactoferrin results in T cell-dependent tumor inhibition of head and neck squamous cell carcinoma in vivo. Int J Cancer. 111(3):398-403.

Ward PP, Paz E, Conneely OM. 2005. Multifunctional roles of lactoferrin: a critical overview. Cell Mol Life Sci. 62(22):2540-8.

Weinberg ED. 2007. Antibiotic properties and applications of lactoferrin. Cur Pharma Design. 13:801-11

Wolf JS, Li G, Varadhachary A, Petrak K, Schneyer M, Li D, Ongkaesuwan M, Zhang X, Taylor RJ, Strome SE, O'Makket BW Jr. 2007. Oral lactoferrin results in T cell-dependent tumor inhibition of head and neck squamous cell carcinoma in vivo. Clin Cancer Res. 13(5):1601-10.

Yamauchi K, Wakabayashi H, Shin K, Takase M. Bovine lactoferrin: benefits and mechanism of action against infections. 2006. Biochem Cell Biol. 84(3):291-6.

Zacharski LR, Ornstein DL, Woloshin S, Schwartz LM. 2000. Association of age, sex, and race with body iron stores in adults: analysis of NHANES III data. Am Heart J. 140(1):98-104.

Zhou JR, Erdman JW Jr. 1995. Phytic acid in health and disease. Crit Rev Food Sci Nutr. 35(6):495-508.

Bibliography

Abalea V, Cillard J, Dubos MP, Anger JP, Cillard P, Morel I. 1998. Iron-induced oxidative DNA damage and its repair in primary rat hepatocyte culture. Carcinogenesis. 19(6):1053-9.

Aessopos A, Kati M, Farmakis D. 2007. Heart disease in thalassemia intermedia: a review of underlying pathophysiology. Hematologica. 92(5):658-65.

Alexander J, Tung BY, Croghan A, Kowdley KV. 2007. Effect of iron depletion on serum markers of fibrogenesis, oxidative stress and serum liver enzymes in chronic hepatitis C: results of a pilot study. Liver Int. 27(2):268-73.

Amit T, Avramovich-Tirosh Y, Youdim MB, Mandel S. 2007. Targeting multiple Alzheimer's disease etiologies with multimodal neuroprotective and neurorestorative iron chelators. FASEB. [Epub ahead of print] PMID: 18048580.

Anderson JK. 2001. Do alterations in glutathione and iron levels contribute to pathology associated with Parkinson's disease? Novartis Found Symp. 235:11-20.

———— 2004. Iron dysregulation and Parkinson's disease. J Alzheimer's Dis. 6(6 Suppl):547-52.

Anderson NE, Sheffield S, Hope JK. 1999. Superficial siderosis of the central nervous system: a late complication of cerebellar tumors. Neurology. 52(1):163-9.

Andrews NC. 1999. Disorders of iron metabolism. N Engl J Med. 341:1986-95.

Antoine D, Braun P, Cervoni P, Schwartz P, Lamy P. 1979. Le cancer bronique des mineurs de fer de Lorraine peut-il étre considoré comme un maladie professionelle? Rev Fr Mal Respir. 7:63-5.

Argyropoulou MI, Metafratzi Z, Kiortsis DN, Bitsis S, Tsatsoulis A, Efremidis S. 2000. T2 relaxation rate as an index of pituitary iron overload in patients with ß-thalassemia major. AJR. 175:1567-1569.

Artym J, Zimecki M, Paprocka M, Kruzel ML. 2003. Orally adminis-tered lactoferrin restores humoral immune response in immunocompromised mice. Immunol Lett. 89(1):9-15.

Asare GA, Bronz M, Naidoo V, Kew MC. 2007. Interactions between aflatoxin B1 and dietary iron overload in hepatic mutagenesis. Toxicology. 234(3):157-66.

Asare GA, Mossanda KS, Kew MC, Peterson AC, Kahler-Venter CP, Siziba K. 2006a. Hepatocellular carcinoma caused by iron overload: a pos-sible mechanism of direct hepatocarcinogenicity. Toxicology 219(1-3):41-52.

Asare GA, Paterson AC, Kew MC, Khan S, Mossanda KS. 2006b. Iron-free neoplastic nodules and hepatocellular carcinoma without cirrho-sis in Wistar rats fed a diet high in iron. J Pathol. 208(1):82-90.

Aust A, Lund L, Chao C, Park S, Fang R. 2000. Role of iron in cellular effects of asbestos. Inhalation Toxicol. 12:S75S-80S.

Avunduk AM, Yardimci S, Avunduk MC, Kurnaz, L, Cengiz M. 2000. A possible mechanism of X-ray-induced injury to the lens. Jpn J Ophthal-mol. 44(1):88-91.

Babbs CF. 1990. Free radicals and the etiology of colon cancer. Free Radic Biol Med. 8(2):191-200.

Bacon BR, Britton RS. 1989. Hepatic injury in chronic iron overload. Role of lipid peroxidation. Chem Biol Interact. 70(3-4):183-226.

Bacon BR, O'Neill R, Britton RS. 1993. Hepatic mitochondrial en-ergy production in rats with chronic iron overload. Gastroenterology. 105(4):1134-40.

Bacon BR. 1997. Iron and hepatitis C. Gut. 41:127-8.

Baird WH, Hooven LA, Mahadevan B. 2005. Carcinogenic polycyclic aromatic hydrocarbon-DNA adducts and mechanism of action. Environ Mol Mutagen. 45(2-3):106-14.

Balder HF, de Vogel J, Jansen MCJf, Weijenberg MP, van den Brandt, PA, Westenbrink S, van der Meer R, Goldbohm RA. 2006. Heme and chlo-rophyll intake and risk of colorectal cancer in the Netherlands cohort study. Cancer Epidemiol Biomarkers Prev. 15(4):717-25.

Baldys A, Aust AE. 2005. Role of iron in inactivation of epidermal growth factor receptor after asbestos treatment of human lung and pleural target cells. Am J Resp Cell Molecular Biol. (32):436-42.

Ball BR, Smith KR, Vernath JM, Aust AE. 2000. Bioavailability of iron from coal fly ash: mechanisms of mobilization and of biological effects. Inhal Toxicol. 12(Suppl 4):209-25.

Barton AL, Banner BR, Cable EE, Bonkovsky HL. 1995. Distribution of iron in the liver predicts the response of chronic hepatitis C infection to interferon therapy. Am J Clin Pathol. 103:419-24.

Bartzokis G, Cummings J, Perlman S, Hance DB, Mintz J. 1999. Increased basal ganglia iron levels in Huntington disease. Arch Neurol. 56(5):569-74.

Bartzokis G, Tishler TA, Shin IS, Lu PH, Cummingl JL. 2004 Brain ferritin iron as a risk factor for age at onset in neurodegerative diseases. Ann N Y Acad Sci. 1012:221-36.

Bartzokis G, Tishler TA. 2000. MRI evaluation of basal ganglia ferritin iron and neurotoxicity in Alzheimer's and Huntington's disease. Cell Mol Biol (Noisy-le-grand). 46(4):821-33.

Başar I, Ayhan A, Bircan K, Ergen A, Taşar C. 1991. Transferrin receptor activity as a marker in transitional cell carcinoma of the bladder. Br J Urol. 67(2):165-8.

Bates DE. 2003. Aminoglycoside ototoxicity. Drugs Today (Barc). 39(4):277-85.

Benhar M, Engelberg D, Levitzki A. 2002. ROS, stress-activated kinases and stress signaling in cancer. EMBO Rep. 3:420-25.

Ben-Shachar D, Eshel G, Finberg JP, Youdim MB. 1991. The iron chelator desferrioxamine (Desferal) retards 6-hydroxydopamine-induced degeneration of nigrostriatal dopamine neurons. J Neurochem. 56(4):1441-4.

Ben-Shachar D, Eshel G, Riederer P, Youdim MB. 1992. Role of iron and iron chelation in dopaminergic-induced neurodegeneration: implication for Parkinson's disease. Ann Neurol. 32 Suppl:S105-10.

Ben-Shachar D, Riederer P, Youdim MB. 1991. Iron-melanin interaction and lipid peroxidation: implications for Parkinson's disease. J Neurochem. 57(5):1609-14.

Ben-Shachar D, Youdim MB. 1990. Selectivity of melaninized nigrastriatal dopamine neurons to degeneration in Parkinson's disease may depend on iron-melanin interaction. J Neural Transm Suppl. 29:251-8.

―――― 1991. Intranigral iron injection induces behavioral and biochemical "parkinsonism" in rats. J Neurochem. 57(6):2133-5.

―――― 1993. Iron, melanin and dopamine interaction: relevance to Parkinson's disease. Prog Neuropsychopharmacol Biol Psychiatry. 17(1):139-50.

Bentur Y, Koren G, Tesoro A, Carley H, Olivien N, Freedman MH.

1990. Comparison of deferoxamine pharmacokinetics between asymptomatic thalassemic children and those exhibiting severe neurotoxicity. Clin Pharmacol Ther. 47(4):478-82.

Benz CC, Clarke CA, Moore II, DH. 2003. Geographic excess of estrogen receptor-positive breast cancer. Cancer Epidem, Biomarkers and Prevention. 12:1525-7.

Berg D, Grote C, Rausch WD, Maurer M, Wesemann W, Riederer P, Becker G. 1999. Iron accumulation in the substantia nigra in rats visualized by ultrasound. Ultrasound Med Biol. 25(6):901-4.

Berg D, Hochstrasser H, Schweitzer KJ, Riess O. 2006. Disturbance of iron metabolism in Parkinson's disease – ultrasonography as a biomarker. Neurotox Res. 9(1):1-13.

Bharath S, Hsu M, Kaur D, Rajagopalan S, Anderson JK. 2002. Glutathione, iron and Parkinson's disease. Biochem Pharmacol 64(5-6): 1037-48.

Bissett D, Chaterjee R, Hannon DP. 1991. Chronic ultraviolet radiation-increase in skin iron and the photoprotective effect of topically applied iron chelators. Photochem Photobiol. 54:215-13.

Bissett DL, McBride JF. 1996. Synergistic topical photoprotection by a combination of the iron chelator 2-furlicioxime and sunscreen. Am Acad Dermatol. 35(4):546-9.

Blass JP, Gibson GE. 1991. The role of oxidative abnormalities in the pathophysiology of Alzheimer's disease. Rev Neurol. 147:513.

Blumenthal HT, Lansing AI, Wheeler PA. 1944. Calcification of the media of the human aorta and its relation to intimal arteriosclerosis, ageing, and disease. Amer J Pathol. 20:655.

Bonkovsky HL. 1991. Iron and the liver. Am J Med Sci. 301:32-43.

Bonkovsky HL, Lambrecht RW. 2000. Iron-induced liver injury. Clin Liver Dis. 4(vi-vii):409-29.

Bonkovsky HL, Lambrecht RW, Shan Y. 2003. Iron as a co-morbid factor in nonhemochromatotic liver disease. Alcohol 30(2):137-44.

Borg D. 2006. In vivo detection of iron and neuromelanin by transcranial sonography – a new approach for early detection of substantia nigra damage. PMID: 16755382.

Bothwell TH, Charlton AW, Cook JD, Finch CA. 1979. *Iron Metabolism in Man.* Oxford: Blackwell Scientific Publications.

Boyd JT, Doll R, Faulds JS, Leiper J. 1970. Cancer of the lung in iron ore (hematite) miners. Br J Indust Med. 27:97-105.

Brewer GJ. 2007. Iron and copper toxicity in disease of aging, particularly atherosclerosis and Alzheimer's disease. Exp Biol Med. 232:323-35.

Brittenham GM. 2003. Iron chelators and iron toxicity. Alcohol. 30(2):151-8.

———— The red cell cycle. In Brock JH, Halliday JW, Pippard MG, Powell LW. 1994. *Iron Metabolism in Health and Disease*. London, Philadelphia, Toronto, Sydney, Toyko: W.B. Saunders Company Ltd.

Britton RS, Bacon BR, Recknagel RO. 1987. Lipid peroxidation and associated hepatic organelle dysfunction in iron overload. 45(2-4):207-39.

Britton RS, Bacon BR. 1994. Role of free radicals in liver disease and hepatic fibrosis. Hepatogastroenterology. 41(4):343-8.

Britton RS, Ramm GA, Olynyk J, Singh R, O'Neill R, Bacon BR. 1994. Pathophysiology of iron toxicity. Adv Exp Med Biol. 356:239-53.

Britton RS. 1996. Metal-induced hepatotoxicity. Semin Liver Dis. 16(1):3-12.

Brock JH, Halliday JW, Pippard MG, Powell LW. 1994. *Iron Metabolism in Health and Disease*. London, Philadelphia, Toronto, Sydney, Toyko: W.B. Saunders Company Ltd.

Bullen JJ, Griffiths E, eds. 1987. *Iron and Infection*. Chichester, New York, Brisbane, Toronto, Singapore: John Wiley and Sons.

Campbell JA. 1940. Effects of precipitated silica and of iron oxide on the incidence of primary lung tumors in mice. Br Med J. 2:275-80.

Campbell KA, Bank B, Milgram NW. 1984. Epileptogenic effects of electrolytic lesions in the hippocampus: role of iron deposition. Exp Neurol. 86:506-14.

Carlsson A, Fornstedt B. 1991. Possible mechanism underlying the special vulnerability of dopaminergic neurons. Acta Neurol Scand Suppl. 136:16-18.

Carter RL, Mitchley BC, Roe FJ. 1968. Induction of tumors in mice and rats with ferric sodium gluconate and iron dextran glycerol glycoside. Br J Cancer. 22(3):521-26.

Carter RL. 1969. Early development of injection-site sarcomas in rats: a study of tumours induced by iron-dextran. Br J Cancer. 23(3):559-66.

Case BW, Ip MP, Padilla M, Kleinerman J. 1986. Asbestos effects on superoxide production. An in vitro study of hamster alveolar macrophages. Environ Res. 39(2):299-306.

Castellani RJ, Honda K, Zhu X, Cash AD, Nunomura A, Perry G, Smith MA. 2004. Contribution of redox-active iron and copper to oxidative damage in Alzheimer disease. Ageing Res Rev. 3:319-26.

Castellani RJ, Siedlak SL, Perry G, Smith MA. 2000. Sequestration of iron by Lewy bodies in Parkinson's disease. Acta Neuroathol (Berl). 100(2):111-4.

Cavalieri EL, Rogan EG, Li K, Todorovic R, Ariese F, Jankowiak R, Gruber N, Small GJ. 2005. Identification and quantification of depurinating DNA adducts formed in mouse skin treated with dibenzo[a,l]pyrine (DB[a,l]P) or its metabolites and in rat mammary gland treated with DB[a,l]P. Chem Res Toxicol. 18:976-83.

Cederbaum AI. 1992. Iron and ethanol-induced tissue damage: Generation of reactive oxygen intermediates and possible mechanisms for their role of alcohol liver toxicity. In: *Iron and Human Disease.* Lauffer RB, ed. Boca Raton, Ann Arbor, London, Tokyo: CRC Press, pp. 419-46.

————— 2003. Iron and CYP2E1-dependent oxidative stress and toxicity. Alcohol. 30(2):115-20.

Chandra Mohan KB, Devraj H, Prathiba D, Hara Y, Nagini S. 2006a. Antiproliferative apoptosis inducing effect of lactoferrin and black tea polyphenol combination on hamster buccal pouch carcinogenesis. Biochim Biophys Acta. 1760(10):1536-44.

Chandra Mohan KB, Kumaraguruparan R, Prathiba D, Nagini S. 2006b. Modulation of xenobiotic-metabolizing enzymes and redox status during chemoprevention of hamster buccal carcinogenesis by bovine lactoferrin. Nutrition. 22(9):940-6.

Chandra RK. 1965. The risk of sarcomatous change after iron-dextran therapy. Indian J Pediatr. 32:75-7.

Chang EF, Claus CP, Vreman HJ, Wong RJ, Noble-Haeusslein LJ. 2005. Heme regulation in traumatic brain injury: relevance to adult and developing brain. J Cerebral Blood Flow & Metab. 25:1401-17.

Chao A, Thun MJ, Connell CJ, McCullough ML, Jacobs EJ, Flanders WD, Rodriguez C, Sinha R, Calle EE. 2005. Meat consumption and risk of colorectal cancer. JAMA. 293(2):233-4.

Chao CC, Lund LG, Zinn KR, Aust AE. 1994. Iron mobilization from crocidolite asbestos by human lung carcinoma cells. Arch Biochem Biophys. 314(2):384-91.

Chao CC, Park SH, Aust AE. 1996. Participation of nitric oxide and iron in the oxidation of DNA in asbestos-treated human lung epithelial cells. Arch Biochem Biophys. 326(1):152-7.

Chau LY. 2000. Iron and atherosclerosis. Proc Natl Sci Repub China B. 24(4):151-5.

Chen Y, Wang J, Huang W. 1999. [Desferrioxamine protects against getamicin ototoxicity]. Zhonghua Er Bi Yan Hou Ke Za Zhi. 34(3):154-6. [In Chinese]

Cheung PT. 2007. Iron, sense and neurotoxicity. Hong Kong Med J. 13(5):412.

Choi JY, Neuhouser ML, Barnett M, Hong CC, Kristal AR, Thornquist M, King IB, Goodman G, Ambrosone CB. 2008. Iron Intake, oxidative stress-related genes (MnSOD and MPO), and prostate cancer risk in CARET cohort. Carcinogenesis. Feb 22 [Epub ahead of print]

Chua-anusorn W, Webb J, Macey DJ, de la Motte, Hall P, St Pierre TG. 1999. The effect of prolonged iron loading on the chemical form of iron oxide deposits in rat liver and spleen. Biochim Biophys Acta. 1454(2):191-200.

Churg A, Hobson J, Berean K, Wright J. 1989. Scavengers of active oxygen species prevent cigarette smoke-induced asbestos fiber penetration in rat tracheal explants. Am J Pathol. 135(4):599-603.

Chwiej J, Adamek D, Szczerbowska-Boruchowska M, Krygowska-Wajs A, Wojcik S Falenberg G, Manka A, Lankosz M. 2007. Investigations of differences in iron oxidation state inside single neurons from substantia nigra of Parkinson's disease and control patients using the micro-XANES technique. J Biol Inorg Chem. 12(2)204-11.

Cohen G. 1984. Oxy-radical toxicity in catecholamine neurons. Neurotoxicology. 5(1)77-82.

Collins MA, Neafsey EJ. 2002. Potential neurotoxic "agents provocateurs" in Parkinson's disease. Neurotoxidol Teratol. 24(5):571-7.

Conlon BJ, Perry BP, Smith DW. 1998. Attenuation of neomycin ototoxicity by iron chelation. Laryngoscope. 108(2):284-7.

Connor JR, Menzies SL, St. Martin S, Fine RE, Mufson EJ. 1991. Altered cellular distribution of transferrin, ferritin and iron in Alzheimer's disease brains. J Neurosci Res. 31:75.

Connor JR, Menzies SL, St Martin SM, Mufson EJ. 1992a. A histochemical study of iron, transferrin, and ferritin in Alzheimer's diseased brains. J Neurosci Res. 31(1):75-83.

Connor JR, Snyder BS, Beard JL, Fine RE, Mufson EJ. 1992b. The regional distribution of iron and iron regulatory proteins in the brain in aging and Alzheimer's disease. J Neurosci Res. 31:327.

Connor JR. 1992. Proteins of iron regulation in the brain in Alzheimer's disease. In Lauffer RB, ed. 1992. *Iron and Human Disease.* Boca Raton, Ann Arbor, London, Tokyo: CRC Press, pp 54-67.

Conway K, Parrish E, Edmiston SN, Tolbert D, Tse C-K, Moorman P, Newman B, Millikan RC. 2007. Risk factors for breast cancer characterized by the estrogen receptor alpha A908G (K303R) mutation. Breast Cancer Research. 9:R36 (Available online at http://breast-cancer-research.com/content/9/3/R36)

Craelius W, Migdal MW, Luessenhop CP, Sugar A, Mihalakis I. 1982. Iron deposits surrounding multiple sclerosis plaques. Arch Pathol Lab Med. 106:397-99.

Crawford R. 2000. *The Iron Elephant*. Glyndon, MD: Vida Publishing, Inc.

Crosby WH. 1986. Yin, yang and iron. Nutrition Today. July/Aug:14-16.

Cross AJ, Gunter MJ, Wood RJ, Pietinen P, Taylor PR, Virtamo J, Albanes D, Sinha R. 2006. Iron and colorectal cancer risk in the alpha-tocopherol, beta-carotene cancer prevention study. Int J Cancer. 118(12):147-52.

Cross AJ, Sinha R. 2004. Meat-related mutagens/carcinogens in the etiology of colorectal cancer. Environ Mol Mutagen. 44(1):44-55.

Crowley JD, Still WJ. 1960. Metastatic carcinoma at the site of injection of iron-dextran complex. Br Med J. 1(5183):1411-12.

Cui Y, Vogt S, Olson N, Glass AG, Rohan TE. 2007. Levels of zinc, selenium, calcium, and iron in benign breast tissue and risk of subsequent breast cancer. 16(8):2173.

Cutler P. 1994. Iron overload an psychiatric illness. Can J Psychiatry. 39:8-11.

Cyrus-David MS, Strom SS. 2001. Chemoprevention of breast cancer with selective estrogen receptor modulators: views from broadly diverse focus groups of women with elevated risk for breast cancer. Psychooncology. 10(6):521-33.

D'Archivio MD, Filesi C, Di Benedetto R, Gargiulo R. 2007. Polyphenols, dietary sources and bioavailability. Ann Ist Super Sanita. 43(4):348-61.

Dai K. Koam K. Bpsland M, Frenkel K, Bernhardt G, Huang X. 2007. Roles of hormone replacement therapy and iron in proliferation of breast epithelial cells with different estrogen and progesterone receptor status. Breast. Oct. 8; [Epub ahead of print].

De Feo TM, Fargion S, Duca L, Cesana BM, Boncinelli L, Lozza P, Cappellini MD, Fiorelli G. 2001. Non-transferrin-bound iron in alcohol abusers. Alcohol Clin Exp Res. 25(10):1494-9.

Deugnier Y, Loréal O, Carré F, Duvallet A, Zoulin F, Vinel JP, Paris

JC, Blaison D, Moirand R, Turlin B, Gandon Y, David V, Mégret A, Guinot M. 2002. Increased body iron stores in elite road cyclists. Med Sci Sports Exerc. 34(5):876-80.

Deugnier Y, Turlin B. 2001. Iron and hepatocellular carcinoma. J Gastroenterol Hepatol. 16(5):491-4.

————— 2002. Iron overload disorders. Clin Liv Dis. 6(2):481-96.

————— 2007. Pathology of hepatic iron overload. World J Gastroenterol. 13(35):4755-4760.

Deugnier Y. 2003. Iron and liver cancer. Alcohol. 30(2):145-50.

Dexter DT, Wells FR, Lees AJ, Agid F, Agid Y, Jenner P, Marsden CD. 1989. Increased nigral iron content and alterations in other metal ions occurring in brain in Parkinson's disease. J Neurochem. 52:1830-6.

Dexter DT, Carayon A, Javoy-Agid F, Agid Y, Wells FR, Daniel SE, Lees AJ, Jenner P, Marsden CD. 1991 Alterations in the levels of iron, ferritin and other trace metals in Parkinson's disease and other neurodegenerative diseases affecting the basal ganglia. Brain. 114:1953-75.

Dey A, Cederbaum AL. 2006. Alcohol and oxidative liver injury. Hepatology. 43:S63-S74.

Distante S, Bjoro K, Hellum KB, Myrvang B, Berg JP, Skaug K, Raknerud N, Bell H. 2002. Raised serum ferritin predicts non-response to interferon and ribavirin treatment in patients with chronic hepatitis C infection. Liver 22(3):269-75.

Dobson J. 2004. Magnetic iron compounds in neurological disorders. Ann NY Acad Sci. 1012:183-92.

Donaldson K, Cullen RT. 1984. Chemiluminescence of asbestos-activated macrophages. Br J Exp Pathol. 65(1):81-90.

Donaldson K, Slight J, Hannant D, Bolton RE. 1985. Increased release of hydrogen peroxide and superoxide anion from asbestos-primed macrophages. Effect of hydrogen peroxide on the functional activity of alpha 1-protease inhibitor. Inflammation. 9(2):139-47.

Doreswami K, Muralidhara. 2005. Genotoxic consequences associated with oxidative damage in testis of mice subjected to iron intoxication. Toxicology. 206(1):169-78.

Double KL, Ben-Shacar D, Youdim MB, Zecca I, Riederer P, Gerlach M. 2002. Influence of neuromelanin on oxidative pathways within the human substantia nigra. Neurotoxicol Teratol. 24(5):621-8.

Double KL, Gerlach M, Schuneman V, Trautwein AX, Zecca L, Gallorini M, Youdim MB, Riederer P, Ben-Schacher D. 2003. Iron-binding characteristics of neuromelanin of the human substantia nigra. Biochem

Pharmacol. 66(3): 489-94.

Double KL, Gerlach M, Youdim MB, Riederer P. 2000. Impaired iron homeostasis in Parkinson's disease. J Neural Transm Suppl. 37-58.

Double KL, Riederer PF, Gerlach M. 1999. Role of iron in 6-hydroxy-dopamine neurotoxicity. Adv Neurol. 80:287-96.

Drewinko B, Moskwa P, Reuben J. 1987. Expression of transferrin receptors is unrelated to proliferative status in cultured human colon cancer cells. Anticancer Res. 7(2):139-41.

Dreyfus J. 1936. Lung carcinoma among siblings who have inhaled dust containing iron oxides during their youth. Clin Med. 30:256-60.

Drobni P, Näslund J, Evander M. 2004. Lactoferrin inhibits human papilomavirus binding and uptke in vitro. Antiviral Res. 64(1):63-8.

Dunaief JL. 2006. Iron induced oxidative damage as a potential factor in age-related macular degeneration: the Cogan Lecture. Invest Ophthalmol Vis Sci. 47:4660-664.

Dunkel VC, San RH, Seifried HE, Whittaker P. 1999. Genotoxicity of iron compounds in Salmonella typhimurium and L5178Y mouse lymphoma cells. Environ Mol Mutagen. 33(1):28-41.

Dunne JR, Gannon CJ, Osborn TM, Taylor MD, Maione DL, Napolitano LM. 2002. Preoperative anemia in colon cancer: assessment of risk factors. Am Surg. 68(6):582-7.

Ebadu NM, Srinivasan SK, Baxi MD. 1996. Oxidative stress and antioxidant therapy in Parkinson's disease. Prog Neurobiol. 48(1):1-19.

Edling C. 1982. Lung cancer and smoking in a group of iron ore miners. Am J Indust Med. 3:191-99.

Eichbaum Q, Foran S, Dziks S. 2003. Is iron gluconate really safer than iron dextran? Blood. 101(9):3756-7.

Ekor M, Farombi EO, Emerole GO. 2006. Modulation of hentamicin-induced renal dysfunction and injury by phenolic extract of soybean (Glycine Max). Fundam Clin Pharmacol. 20(3):263-71.

Elliott RL, Elliott MC, Wang F, Head JF. 1993. Breast carcinoma and the role of iron metabolism. A cytochemical, tissue culture, and ultrastructural study. Ann NY Acad Sci. 698:159-66.

Elstner EF, Schultz W, Vogl G. 1988. Cooperative stimulation by sulfite and crocidolite asbestos fibers on enzyme catalyzed production of reactive oxygen species. Arch Toxicol. 62(6):424-7.

Elstner EF. Schütz W, Vogl G. 1986. Enhancement of enzyme-catalyzed production of reactive oxygen species by suspensions of "crocidolite" asbestos fibres. Free Radic Res Commun. 1(6):355-9.

Emery T, Neilands JB. 1961. Structure of the ferrichrome compounds. J Am Chem Soc. 83:1626.

Emery TF. 1991. *Iron and Your Health: Facts and Fallacies.* Boca Raton, Ann Arbor, London, Tokyo: CRC Press.

English DR, MacInnis RJ, Hodge AM, Hopper JL, Haydon AM, Giles GG. 2004. Red meat, chicken, and fish consumption and risk of colorectal cancer. Cancer Epidemiol Biomarkers Prev. 2004. 13(9):1509-14.

Enochs WS, Sarna T, Zecca L, Swatz HM. 1994. The roles of neuromelanin, binding of metal ions, and oxidative cytotoxicity in the pathogenesis of Parkinson's disease: a hypothesis. J Neural Transm Park Dis Dement Sect. 7(2): 83-100.

Erdemoglu AK, Ozbakir S. 2002. Serum ferritin levels and early prognosis of stroke. Eur J Neurol. 9(6):633-7.

Esiri MM, Taylor CR, Mason DY. 1976. Applications of an immunoperoxidase method to a study of the central nervous system: Preliminary findings in a study of human formalin-fixed material. Neuropathol Appl Neurobiol. 2:233-46.

Facchini FS. 2002. *The Iron Factor of Aging. Why Do Americans Age Faster?* Tucson, AZ: Fenestra Books.

Fahn S, Cohen G. 1992. The oxidant stress hypothesis in Parkinson's disease: evidence supporting it. Ann Neurol. 32(6):804-12.

Fang R, Aust AE. 1997. Induction of ferritin synthesis in human lung epithelial cells treated with crocidolite asbestos. Arch Biochem Biophys. 340(2):369-75.

Fargion S, Fracanzani AL, Romano R, Cappellini MD, Faré M, Mattioli M, Piperano A, Ronchi G, Fiorelli G. 1996. Genetic hemochromatosis in Italian patients with porphyria cutanea tarda: possible explanation for iron overload. Hepatol. 24(5):564-9.

Fargion S, Fracanzani AL, Sampietro M, Molteni V, Boldorini R, Mattioli M, Cesana B, Lunghi G, Piperno A, Valsecchi C, Fiorelli G. 1997. Liver iron influences the response to interferon alpha therapy in chronic hepatitis C. Eur J Gastroenterol Hepatol. 9(5):497-503.

Faucheux BA, Hirsch BC. 1998. [Iron homeostasis and Parkinson's disease.] Ann Biol Clin (Paris). 56 Spec No: 23-30. [French]

Faucheux BA, Martin ME, Beaumont C, Hauw JJ, Agrid Y, Hirsch BC. 2003. Neuromelanin associated redox-active iron is increased in the substantia nigra of patients with Parkinson's disease. J Neurochem. 86(5): 1142-8.

FDA. 1997. Iron-Containing Supplements and Drugs: Label Warning Statements and Unit-Dose Packaging Requirements. Federal Register 62 FR 2217.

Feder JN, Gnirke A, Thomas Z, Tsuchihashi Z, Ruddy DA, Basava A, Dormishian G, Domingo R Jr, Ellis MC, Fullan A, Hinton LM, Jones NL, Kimmel BE, Kronmal GS, Lauer P, Lee VK, Loeb DB, Mapa FA, McClelland E, Meyer NC, Mintier GA, Moeller N, Moore T, Morikang EB, Prass CE, Quintana L, Stames SM, Schatzman RC, Brunke KJ, Drayana DT, Risch NJ, Bacon BR, Wolff RK. 1996. A novel MHC class 1-like gene is mutated in patients with hereditary haemochromatosis. Nat Genet. 13(4):399-408.

Feelders RA, Vreugdenhil G, Eggermont AM, Kuiper-Kramer PA, van Ejk HG, Swaak AJ. 1998. Regulation of iron metabolism in the acute-phase response: interferon gamma and tumour necrosis factor alpha induce hypoferraemia, ferritin production and a decrease in circulating transferrin receptors in cancer patients. Eur J Clin Invest. 28(7):520-7.

Ferrali M, Signorini C, Sugherini L, Pompella A, Lodovici M, Caciotti B, Camporti M. 1997. Release of free, redox-active iron in the liver and DNA oxidative damage following phenylhydrazine intoxication. Biochem Pharmacol. 53(11):1743-51.

Ferré, C. 1997. *Pocket Guide to Macrobiotics*. Berkeley, CA: Crossing Press.

Ferré, J. 2007. *Basic Macrobiotic Cooking: Twentieth Anniversary Edition*. Chico, CA: George Ohsawa Macrobiotic Foundation.

Finch SC, Finch CA. 1955. Medicine (Baltimore). 34:384-430.

Fleming DJ, Tucker KL, Jacques PR, Dallal GE, Wilson PWF, Wood RJ. 2002. Dietary factors associated with the risk of high iron stores in the elderly Framingham Heart Study cohort. Am J Clin Nutr. 76:1375-84.

Fletcher LM, Bridle KR, Crawford DH. 2003. Effect of alcohol on iron storage diseases of the liver. Best Pract Res Clin Gastroenterol. 17(4):663-77.

Fletcher LM, Powell LW. 2003. Hemochromatosis and alcoholic liver disease. Alcohol. 30(2):131-6.

Floor E. 2000. Iron as a vulnerability factor in nigrostriatal degeneration in aging and Parkinson's disease. Cell Mol Biol (Noisy-le-grand). 46(4): 709-20.

Food and Nutrition Board. 1993. *Iron Deficiency Anemia: Recommended Guidelines for the Prevention, Detection, and Management Among U.S. Children and Women of Childbearing Age*. Earl R, Woteki CE, eds.

Washington, DC: National Academy Press.

Food and Nutrition Board. 2001. *Dietary Reference Intakes for Vitamin A, Vitamin K, Arsenic, Boron, Chromium, Copper, Iodine, Iron, Manganese, Molybdenum, Nickel, Silicon, Vanadium, and Zinc.* Washington, DC: National Academy Press.

Fujita N, Horiike S, Sugimoto R, Tanaka H, Iwasa M, Kobayashi Y, Hasegawa K, Ma N, Kawanishi S, Adachi Y, Kaito M. 2007a. Hepatic oxidative DNA damage correlates with iron overload in chronic hepatitis C patients. 42(3):353-62.

Fujita N, Sugimoto R, Urawa N, Araki J, Mifuji R, Yamamoto M, Horiike S, Tanaka H, Iwasa M, Kobayashi Y, Adachi Y, Kaito M. 2007b. Hepatic iron accumulation is associated with disease progression and resistance to interferon/ribavirin combination therapy in chronic hepatitis C. J Gastroenterol Hepatol. 22(11):1886-93.

Furst A. 1960. Metals in tumors. In: *Metal Binding in Medicine.* Steven MJ, Johnson LA, eds. Philadelphia: J B Lippincott, p. 346.

Furutani T, Hino K, Okuda M, Gondo T, Nishina S, Kitase A, Korenaga M, Xiao SY, Weinman SA, Lemon SM, Sakaida I, Okita K. 2006. Hepatic iron overload induces hepatocellular carcinoma in transgenic mice expressing the hepatitis C virus polyprotein. Gastroenterology. 130(7):2087-98.

Gackowski D, Kruszewski M, Banaszkiewicz Z, Jawien A, Olinski R. 2002. Lymphocyte labile iron pool, plasma iron, transferrin saturation and ferritin levels in colon cancer parients. Acta Biochimica Polonica. 49 1:269-72.

Gal S, Fridkin M, Amit T, Aheng H, Youdim MB. 2006. M30, a novel multifunctional neuroprotective drug with potent iron chelating and brain selective monoamine oxidase-ab inhibitory activity for Parkinsonson's disease. Neural Transm Suppl. 70:447-56.

Galazka-Friedman J, Friedman A. 1997. Controversies about iron in parkinsonian and control substantia nigra. Acta Neurobiol Exp (Wars). 57(3):217-225.

Galey JB, Destrée O, Dumats J, Gébard S, Tachon P. 2000. Protection against oxidative damage by iron chelators: effect of lipophilic analogues and prodrugs of N,N-bis(3,4,5-trimethoxylbenzyl) ethylene-diamine N,N-diacetic acid (OR10141). J Med Chem. 43:1418-21.

Garcon G, Gosset P, Maunit B, Zerimech F, Creusy C, Muller JF, Shirall P. 2004a. Influence of iron ($^{56}Fe_2O_3$ or $^{54}Fe_2O_3$) in the upregulation of chtochrome P4501A1 by benzo[a]pyrene in the respiratory tract of Sprague-Dawley rats. App. Toxicol. 24(3):249-56.

Garcon G, Gosset P, Zerimech F, Grave-Descampiaux B, Shirali P. 2004b. effect of Fe_2O_3on the capacity of benzo[a]pyrene to induce polycyclic aromatic hydrocarbon-metabolizind enzymes in the respiratory tract of Sprague-Dawley rats. Toxicol Lett. 150(2):179-89.

Garrison C, ed. 2001. *Iron Disorders Institute Guide to Hemochromatosis.* Nashville, TN: Cumberland House.

——— 2003. *The Iron Disorders Institute Guide to Anemia.* Nashville, TN: Cumberland House.

——— 2005. *Exposing the Hidden Dangers of Iron.* By Weinberg ED. Nashville, TN: Cumberland House.

Garrison C, Rasswater A. 2008. *The Hemochromatosis Cookbook: Recipes and Menus for Reducing the Iron in Your Diet.* Nashville, TN: Cumberland House.

Gelman BB, Rodriguz-Wolf MS, Wen J. 1992. Siderotic cerebral macrophages in aquired immunodeficiency syndrome. Arch Pathol Lab Med. 116:509.

Gerlach M, Bouble KL, Ben-Shachar D, Zecca L, Youdim MB, Riederer P. 2003. Neuromelanin and its interaction with iron as a potential risk factor for dopaminergic neurodegeneration underlying Parkinson's disease. Neurotox Res. 5(1-2):35-44.

Giler S, Moroz C. 1978. The significance of ferritin in malignant diseases. Biomedicine. 28(4):203-6.

Gillie A. 1964. Iron-dextran and sarcomata. Br Med J. 1(5398):1593-4.

Giovannini C, Scazzocchio B, Vari R, Santangelo C, D'Achivio M, Masella R. 2007. Apoptosis in cancer and atherosclerosis: polyphenol activities. Ann Ist super Sanita, 43(4):406-16.

Giuffrida G, Condorelli M, Filocamo G Jr, Migliau G, Pugliese F, Basile U. 1964. Carcinogenic risk of iron-dextran. Br Med J. 1(5398):1583-4.

Gloyne SR. 1935. Two cases of squamous carcinoma of the lung occurring in asbestosis. Tubercle. 17:5-10.

Gocht A, Lohler J. 1990. Changes in glial cell markers in recent and old demyelating lesions in central pontine myelinolysis. Acta Neuropathol. 80:46-58.

Good PF, Olanow CW, Perl DP. 1992. Neuromelanin-containing neurons of the substantia nigra accumulate iron and aluminum in Parkinson's disease; a LAMMA study. Brain res. 593(2):343-6.

Goodglick LA, Kane AB. 1986. Role of reactive oxygen metabolites in crocidolite asbestos toxicity to mouse macrophages. Cancer Res.

46(11):5558-66.

Goodglick LA, Kane AB. 1990. Cytotoxicity of long and short crocidolite asbestos fibers in vitro and in vivo. Cancer Res. 50(16):5153-63.

Goodman L. 1953. Alzheimer's disease: a clinoco-pathologic analysis of twenty-three cases with a theory on pathogenesis. J Nerv Ment Dis. 118:97.

Gotz ME, Freyberger A, Riederer P. 1990. Oxidative stress: a role in the pathogenesis of Parkinson's disease. J Neural Transm Suppl. 29:241-9.

Graf E, Eaton JW. 1990. Antioxidant functions of phytic acid. Free Radic Biol Med. 8(1):61-9.

Graf E, Empsos KL. 1987. Phytic acid: a natural antioxidant. JBC. 262(24):11647-50.

Griffiths E, Bullen JJ. 1987. Iron-binding proteins and host defense. In: *Iron and Infection.* Chichester, New York, Brisbane, Toronto, Singapore: John Wiley and Sons, pp 171-211.

Griffiths PD, Crossman AR. 1993. Distribution of iron in the basal ganglia and neocortex in postmortem tissue in Parkinson's disease and Alzheimer's disease. Dementia. 4(2):61-5.

Grotto HZ. 2008. Anaemia of cancer: an overview of mechanisms involved in its pathogenesis. Med Oncol. 25(1):12-21.

Grunblatt E, Mandel S, Youdim MB. 2000. Neuroprotective strategies in Parkinson's disease using the models of 6-hydroxydopamine and MPTP. Ann N Y Acad Sci. 899:262-73.

Guggenbuhl P, Deugnier Y, Boisdet JF, Rolland Y, Perdriger A, Pawlotsky Y, Chalds G. 2005. Bone mineral densiry in men with genetic hemochromatosis and HFE gene mutation. Osteoporos Int. 16(12):1809-14.

Gunel-Ozcan A, Alyilmaz-Bekmez , Guler EN, Guc D. 2006. HFE H63D mutation frequency shows an increae in Turkish women with breast cancer. BMC Cancer. 6:37.

Guo WD, Chow WH, Zheng W, Li JY, Blot WJ. 1994. Diet, serum markers and breast cancer mortality in Chiona. Jpn J Cancer Res. 85(6):572-7.

Gura T. 1999. New genes boost rice nutrients. Science. 285:994-5.

Haddow A, Horning ES. 1960. On the carcinogenicity of an iron-dextran complex. J Natl Cancer Inst. 24:109-47.

Haddow A, Roe FJ, Mitchley BC. 1964. Induction of sarcomata in rabbits by intramuscular injection of iron-dextran ("Imferon"). Br Med J. 1(5398):1593-4.

Hall S, Rutledge JN, Schallert T. 1992. MRI, brain iron and experimental Parkinson's disease. J Neurol Sci. 113(2):198-208.

Halliwell B, Gutteridge JMC. 1984. Oxygen toxicity, oxygen radicals, transition metals and disease. Biochem J. 219:1.

Halliwell B, Zhao K, Whiteman M. 2000. The gastrointestinal tract: a major site of antioxidant action? Free Radic Res. 33(6):819-30.

Han J, Cheng FC, Yang Z, Dryhurst G. 1999. Inhibitors of mitochondrial respiration, Iron (II), and hydroxyl radical evoke release and extracellular hydrolysis of glutathione in the rat striatum and substantia nigra: potential implications to Parkinson's disease. J Neurochem. 73(4): 1683-95.

Hansen K, Mossman BT. 1987. Generation of superoxide (O_2^-) from alveolar macrophages exposed to asbestiform and nonfibrous particles. Cancer Res. 47(6):1681-6.

Hardy JA, Aust AE. 1995. The effect of iron binding on the ability of crocidolite asbestos to catalyze DNA single-strand breaks. Carcinogenesis. 16(2):319-25.

Harrison-Findik DD, Schafer D, Klein E, Timchenko NA, Kulaksiz H, Clemens D, Fein E, Andropoulos B, Pantopoulos K, Gollan J. 2006. Alcohol metabolism-mediated oxidative stress down-regulates hepcidin transcription and leads to increased duodenal iron transporter expression. J Biol Chem. 281(32):22974-82.

Harrison-Findik DD, Klein E, Crist C, Evans J, Timchenko N, Gollan J. 2007. Iron-mediated regulation of liver hepcidin expression in rats and mice is abolished by alcohol. Hepatology. 46(6):1979-85.

Harrison-Findik DD. 2007. Role of alcohol in the regulation of iron metabolism. World J Gastroenterol. 13(37):4925-30.

Hawkins PT, Poyner DR, Jackson TR, Letcher AJ, Lander DA, Irvine RF. 1993. Inhibition of iron-catalysed hydroxyl radical formation by inositos polyphosphates: a possible physiological function for *myo*-inositol hexakisphosphate. Biochem J. 294:929-34.

He X, Hahn P, Iacovelli J, Wong R, King C, Bhisitkul R, Massaro-Giordano M, Dunaief JL. 2007. Progress in Retinal and Eye Research. 26: 649-73.

Hileti D, Panayiotidis P, Hoffbrand AV. 1995. Iron chelators induce apoptosis in proliferating cells. Br J Haematol. 89:181-7.

Hirata I, Hoshimoto M, Saito O, Kayazawa M, Nishikawa T, Murano M, Toshina K, Wang FY, Matsuse R. 2007. Usefulness of fecal lactoferrin and hemoglobin in diagnosis of colorectal disease. World J Gastroenterol. 13(10):1569-74.

Hirsch EC. 1993. Does oxidative stress participate in nerve cell death in Parkinson's disease? Eur Neurol. 33 Suppl 1:52-9.

―――― 2006. Altered regulation of iron transport and storage in Parkinson's disease. J Neural Transm Suppl. 71: 201-4.

―――― 1994. Biochemistry of Parkinson's disease with special reference to the dopaminergic systems. Mol Neurobiol. 9(1-3): 135-42.

Honda K, Casadesus G, Petersen RB, Perry G, Smith MA. 2004. Oxidative stress and redox-active iron in Alzheimer's disease. Ann N Y Acad Sci 1012:179-82.

Hong CC, Ambrosone CB, Ahn J, Choi JY, McCullough ML, Stevens VL, Rodriguez C, Thun MJ, Calle EE. 2007. Genetic variability in iron-related oxidative stress pathways (Nrf2, NQ01, NOS3. and OH-1), iron intake and risk of postmenopausal breast cancer. Cancer Epidemiol Biomarkers Prev. 16(9):1784-94.

Hua Y, Keep RF, Hoff, JT, Xi G. 2007. Brain injury after intracerebral hemorrhage. The role of thrombin and iron. Stroke. 38[part 2]:759-62.

Huang X. 2003. Iron overload and its association with cancer risk in humans: evidence for iron as a carcinogenic metal. Mutat Res. 533:153-71.

Hughes JT, Oppenheimer DR. 1969. Superficial siderosis of the central nervous system. A report on nine cases with autopsy. Acta Neuropathol (Berl). 13:56-74.

IARC. 1973. *Some Inorganic and Organomatellic Compounds.* IARC Monographs of the Evaluation of Carcinogenic Risk to Humans. Vol. 2. Lyon France: International Agency for Research on Cancer, p 181.

Icso J, Szollosova M, Sorahan T. 1994. Lung cancer among iron ore miners in east Slovakia: a case-control study. Occup Environ Med. 51:642-3.

Iguchi H, Kojo S. 1989. Possible generation of hydrogen peroxide and lipid peroxidation of erythrocyte membrane by asbestos: cytotoxic mechanism of asbestos. Biochem Int. 18(5):981-90.

Ikeda M. 2001. Iron overload without the C282Y mutation in patients with epilepsy. J Neurol Neurosurg Psychiatry. 70:551-53.

Inoue T, Cavanaugh PG, Steck PA, Brünner N, Nicholson GL. 1993. Differences in transferrin response and numbers of transferrin receptors in rat and human mammary carcinoma lines of different metastatic potentials. J Cell Physiol. 156(1):212-7.

Ioannou GN, Weiss NS, Kowdley KV. 2007. Relationship between transferrin-iron saturation, alcohol consumption, and the incidence of cirrhosis and liver cancer. Clin Gastroenterol Hepatol. 5(5):624-9.

Izumi Y, Sawada H, Sakka N, Yamamoto N, Kume T, Katsuki H, Shimohama S, Akaike A. 2005. p-Quinone mediates 6-hydroxydopamine-induced dopaminergic neuronal death and ferrous iron accelerates the conversion of p-quinone into melanin extracellularly. J Neurosci Res 79(6):849-60.

Jacobs A, Jones B, Ricketts C, Bulbrook RD, Wang DY. 1976. Serum ferritin concentration in early breast cancer. Br J Cancer. 34(3):286-90.

Jellinger K, Kienzl E, Rumpelmair G, Riederer P, Stachelberger H, Ben-Shachar D, Youdin MB. 1992. Iron-melanin complex in substantia nigra of parkinsonian brains: an x-ray microanalysis. J Neurochem. 59(3):1168-71.

Jellinger K, Paulus W, Guundke-Iqbal I, Riederer P, Youdim MB. 1990. Brain iron ferritin in Parkinson's and Alzheimer's disease. J Neural Transm Park Dis Dement Sect.2(4):327-40.

Jellinger KA. 1999. The role of iron in neurodegeneration: prospects for pharmacotherapy of Parkinson's disease. Drugs Aging. 14(2):115-40.

Jenner P, Olanow CW. 1996. Oxidative stress and the pathogenesis of Parkinson's disease. Neurology. 47(6 Suppl 3):S161-70.

Jenner P, Schapira AH, Marsden CD. 1992. New insights into the cause of Parkinson's disease. Neurology. 42(12):2241-50.

Jenner P. 1989. Clues to the mechanism underlying dopamine cell death in Parkinson's disease. J Neurol Neurosurg Psychiatry. Suppl:22-8.

——— 1991. Oxidative stress as a cause of Parkinson's disease. Acta Neurol Scand Suppl. 136:6-15.

——— 1992. What process causes nigral cell death in Parkinson's disease? Neurol Clin. 10(2):387-403.

——— 1993. Altered mitochondrial function, iron metabolism and glutathione levels in Parkinson's disease. Acta Neurol Scand Suppl. 146:6-13.

——— 1993. Presymptomatic detection of Parkinson's disease. J Neural Transm Suppl. 40:23-36.

——— 1998. Oxidative mechanisms in nigral cell death in Parkinson's disease. Mov Disord. 13 Suppl 1: 24-34.

Jiang H, Song N, Wang J, Ren Ly, Xie JX. 2007. Peripheral iron dextran induced degeneration of dopaminergic neurons in rat substantia nigra. Neurochem Int. 51(1):32-6.

Jiang R, Manson JAE, Meigs JB, Ma Jing, Rifai N, Hu FB. 2004. Body iron stores in relation to risk of type 2 diabetes in apparently healthy women. JAMA. 291(6):711-17.

Jones HJ, Hedley WE. 1983. Idiopathic hemochromatosis (IHC): dementia and ataxia as presenting signs. Neurology. 33:1479-83.

Kabat GC, Miller AB, Jain M, Rohan TE. 2007. Dietary iron and heme iron intake and risk of breast cancer: a prospective cohort study. Cancer Epidemiol Biomarkers Prev. 16(6):1306-8.

Kabat GC, Rohan TE. 2007. Does excess iron play a role in breast carcinogenesis? an unresolved hypothesis. Cancer Causes Control. 18(10):1047-53.

Kadota K, Wada T, Watatani M, Houjou T, Mori N, Yasutomi M. 1991. [The elevation of serum iron level with oral administration of medoprogesterone acetate (MPA) in patients with brease cancer.] Gan To Kagaku Ryoho. 18(6):983-7. [Article in Japanese]

Kallianpur AR, Hall LD, Yadav M, Christman BW, Dittus RS, Haines JL, Parl FR, Summar ML. 2004. Increased prevalence of the DFE C282Y hemochromatosis allele in women with breast cancer. Cancer Epidemiol Biomarkers Prev. 13:205-12.

Kallianpur AR, Lee SA, Gao YT, Lu W, Zheng Y, Ruan ZX, Dai Q, Gu K, Shu XO, Zheng W. 2008. Dietary animal-derived iron and fat intake and breast cancer risk in the Shanghai Breast Cancer Study. Breast Cancer Res Treat. 107(1):123-32.

Kallianpur AR, Lee SA, Gao YT, Lu W, Zheng ZX, Dai Q, Gu K, Shu XO, Zheng W. 2007. Dietary animal-derived iron and fat intake and breast cancer risk in the Shanghai Breast Cancer Study. Breast Cancer Res Treat. Mar 13. [Epub ahead of print]

Kamp DW, Graceffa P, Pryor WA, Weitzman SA. 1992. The role of free radicals in asbestos-induced diseases. 12(4):293-315.

Kamp DW, Israbian VA, Preusen SE, Zhang CX, Weitzman SA. 1995. Asbestos causes DNA strand breaks in cultured pulmonary epithelial cells: role of iron-catalysed free radicals. Am J Physiol. 268:L471-80.

Kamp DW, Israbian VA, Yeidandi AV, Panos RJ, Graceffa P, Weitzman SA. 1995. Phytic acid, an iron chelator, attenuates pulmonary inflammation and fibrosis in rats after intratracheal instillation of asbestos. Toxicol Pathol. 23(6):689-95.

Kang JO, Jones C, Brothwell B. 1998. Toxicity associated with iron overload found in hemochromatosis: possible mechanism in a rat model. Clin Lab Sci. 11(6):350-4.

Kanwar JR, Palmano KP, Sun X, Kanwar RK, Gupta R, Haggarty N,

Rowan A, Ram S, Krissansen GW. 'Ion-saturated' lactoferrin is a potent natural adjuvant for augmenting cancer chemotherapy. Immunol Cell Biol. [Epub ahead of print].

Kato I, Dnistrian AM, Schwartz M, Toniolo P, Koenig K, Shore RE, Zeleniuch-Jacquotte A, Akhmedkhanov A, Riboli E. 1999. Iron intake, body iron stores and colorectal cancer risk in women: a nested case-control study. Int J Cancer. 80(5):693-8.

Kato J, Miyanishi K, Kobune M, Nakamura T, Takada K, Takimoto R, Kawano Y, Takahashi S, Takahashi M, Sato Y, Takayama T, Niitsu Y. 2007. Long-term phlebotomy with low-iron diet therapy lowers risk of development of hepatocellular carcinoma from chronic hepatitis C. Gastroenterol. 42(10):830-6.

Kaur D, Anderson JK. 2002. Ironing out Parkinson's disease: is therapeutic treatment with iron chelators a real possibility? Aging Cell. 1(1):17-21.

Keer HN, Koziowski JM, Lee C, McEwan RN, Grayhack JT. 1990. Elevated transferrin receptor content in human prostate cancer cell lines assessed in vitro and in vivo. J Urol. 143(2):381-5.

Kew MC, Asare GA. 2007. Dietary overload in the African and hepatocellular carcinoma. 27(6):735-43.

Kienzl E, Jellinger K, Stachelberger H, Linert W. 1999. Iron as a catalyst for oxidative stress in the pathogenesis of Parkinson's disease? Life Sci. 65(18-19):1973-6.

Kienzl E, Puchinger L, Jellinger K, Linert W, Stachelberger H, Jameson RF. 1995. The role of transition metals in the pathogenesis of Parkinson's disease. J Neurol Sci. 134 Suppl: 69-78.

Kitazawa M, Ishitsuka Y, Kobayashi M, Nakano T, Iwasaki K, Sakamoto K Arakane K, Suzuki T, Klingman LH. 2005. Protective effects of an antioxidant derived from serine and vitamin B6 on skin photoaging in hairless mice. Photochem Photobiol. 81:970-4.

Koeppen AH, Barron KD, Csiza CK, Greenfield EA. 1988. Comparative immunocytochemistry of Palizaeus-Merzbacher disease, the jimpy mouse, and the myelin-deficient rat. J Neurol Sci. 84:315-27.

Koerten HD, Brederoo P, Ginsel LA, Daems WT. 1986. The endocytosis of asbestos by mouse peritoneal macrophages and its long-term effect on iron accumulation and labyrinth formation. Eur J Cell Biol. 40(1):25-36.

Koerten HD, Hazekamp J, Kroon M, Daems WT. 1990. Asbestos body formation and iron accumulation in mouse peritoneal granulomas after the introduction of crocidolite asbestos fibers. Am J Pathol. 136(1):141-57.

Kokocińska D, Widala E, Donocik J, Nolewajka E. 1999. [The value of evalualting tumor markers: CA 15-3 and ferritin in blood serum of patients group as "high risk" for breast cancer.] Przegl Lek. 56(10):664-7. [Article in Polish]

Kong S, Davison AJ. 1981. The relative effectiveness of ·OH, H_2O_2, O_2^-, and reducing free radicals in causing damage to biomembranes. A study of radiation damage to erythrocyte ghosts using selective free radical scavengers. Biochem Biophys Acta. 640(1):313-25.

Kong S, Davison AN, Bland J. 1981. Actions of gamma-radiation on resealed erythrocyte ghosts. A Comparison with intact erythrocytes and a study of the effects of oxygen. Int J Radiat Biol Relat Study Phys Chem Med. 40(1):19-29.

Kosano H, Takatani O. 1990. Increase of transferrin binding induced by an alkyl-lysophospholipid in breast cancer cells. J Lipid Mediat. 2(2):117-21.

Krause A, Neitz S, Magert HJ, Schulz A, Forssmann WG, Schula A, Forssmann WG, Schulz-Knappe P, Adermann K. 2000. LEAP-1, a novel highly disulfide-bonded human peptide, exhibits antimicrobial activity. FEBS Lett. 480:147-50.

Krikker MA. 1982. A foundation for hemochromatosis (letter). Ann Intern Med. 97:782-83.

Kucharzewski M, Braziewica J, Majewska U, Gózdz S. 2003. Iron concentrations in intestinal cancer tissue and in colon and rectum polyps. Biol Trace Elem Res. 95(1):19-28.

Kudo H, Suzuki S, Watanabe A, Kikuchi H, Sassa S, Sakamoto S. 2008. Effects of iron overload on renal and hepatic siderosis and the femur in male rats. Toxicology. [Epub ahead of print]

Kunz J. 1964. [Autoradiographic studies on mast cells in iron dextran-induced sarcoma.] Acta Biol Med Ger. 13:233-8. (German)

Kuratko CN. 1998. decrease of manganese superoxide dismutase activity in rats fed high levels of iron during colon carcinogenesis. Food Chem Toxicol. 36(9-10)819-24.

Kushi, A. 1985. *Complete Guide to Macrobiotic Cooking.* New York: Warner Books.

Kushner JP, Lee GR, Macht S. 1972. The role of iron in pathogenesis of porphyria cutanea tarda. J Clin Invest. 51(12):3044-51.

Kvam E, Hejmadi V, Ryter S, Pourzand C, Tyrrell RM. 2000. Heme oxygenase activity causes transient hypersensitivity to oxidative ultraviolet

A radiation that depends on release of iron from heme. Free Radic Biol Med. 28(8):1191-6.

Lai H, Sasaki T, Singh NP. 2005a. Targeted treatment of cancer with artemisinin-tagged iron-carrying compounds. Expert Opin Ther Targets. 9(5):995-1007.9.

Lai H, Sasaki T, Songh NP, Messay A. 2005b. Effects of artemisinin-tagged holotransferin on cancer cells. Life Sci. 76(11):1267-79.

Lange, AE. 2007. The progression of Parkinson disease: a hypothesis. Neurology. 68(2):948-52.

Langston JW. 1988. Neuromelanin-containing neurons are selectively vulnerable in parkinsonism. Trends Pharmacol Sci. 9(10):347-8.

Larsson SC, Rafter J, Holmberg L, Bergkvist L, Wolk A. 2004. Red meat consumption and risk of cancers of the proximal colon, distal colon and rectum: The Swedish Mammography Cohort. Int J Cancer. 113(5):829-34.

———— 2005b. Red meat consumption and risk of cancers of the proximal colon, distal colon and rectum: The Swedish Mammography Cohort. Int J Cancer. 113:829-34.

Larsson SC, Adami HO, Giovannucci E, Wolk A. 2005a. Correspondence. Re: Heme iron, zinc, alcohol consumption, and risk of colon cancer. J Natl Cancer Inst. 97(3):222-233.

Lauffer RB. 1991. *Iron Balance. The New "Iron-Lite" Health Plan that Restores Your Inner Vitality.* New York: St Martin's Press.

———— 1993. *Iron and Your Heart.* New York: St Martin's Press.

Lauffer RB, ed. 1992. *Iron and Human Disease.* Boca Raton, Ann Arbor, London, Tokyo: CRC Press.

Lautermann J, Dehne N, Schacht J, Jahnke K. 2004. [Aminoglycoside- and cisplatin-ototoxicity: from basic science to clinics]. Laryngorhinoot-ologie. 83(5):317-23. [In German]

Lee DH, Anderson KE, Folsom AR, Jacobs DR Jr. 2005a. Heme iron, zinc and upper digestive tract cancer: the Iowa Women's Health Study. Int J Cancer. 117(4):643-7.

Lee DH, Anderson KE, Harnack LJ, Folsom AR, Jacobs DR Jr. 2004a. Heme iron, zinc, alcohol consumption, and colon cancer: Iowa Women's Health Study. J Natl Cancer Inst. 96:403-7.

———— 2004b. Heme iron, zinc, alcohol consumption, and colon cancer: Iowa Women's Health Study. J Natl Cancer Inst. 96(5):403-7.

Lee DH, Jacobs Jr DR, Folsom AR. 2004c. A hypothesis: interaction between supplemental iron intake and fermentation affecting the risk of colon cancer. The Iowa Women's Health Study. 48(1):1-5.

Lee DH, Jacobs DR Jr, Anderson KE. 2005. Correspondence. Response Re: Heme iron, zinc, alcohol consumption, and risk of colon cancer. J Natl Cancer Inst. 97(3):233.

Lee DH, Jacobs DR Jr. 2005 Interaction among heme iron, zinc, and supplemental vitamin C intake on the risk of lung cancer: Iowa Women's Health Study. Nutr Cancer 52(2):130-7.

Lesniak W, Pecoraro VL, Schacht J. 2005. Ternary complexes of gentamicin with iron and lipid catalyzed formation of reactive oxygen species. Chem Res Toxicol. 18(2):357-64.

Levine SM, Chakrabarty A. 2004. The role of iron in the pathogenesis of experimental allergic encephalomyelitis and multiple sclerosis. Ann NY Acad Sci. 1012:252-66.

Li Z, Xia W, Fang B, Yan DH. 2001. Targeting HER-2/neu-overexpressing breast cancer cells by an antisense iron responsive element-directed gene expression. Cancer Let. 174(2):151-8.

Liehr JC, Jones JS. 2001. Role of iron in estrogen-induced cancer. Curr Med Chem. 8(7):839-49.

Loeffler DA, Connor JR, Juneau PL, Snyder BS, Kanaley L, De Maggio AJ, Nguyen H, Brickman CM, LeWitt PA. 1995. Transferrin and iron in normal, Alzheimer's disease, and Parkinson's disease regions. J Neurochem. 66(2):710-24.

Lopez-Barcons LA, Polo D, Liorens A, Reig F, Fabra A. 2005. Targeted adriamycin delivery to MXT-B2 metastatic mammary carcinoma cells by transferrin liposomes: effecxt of adriamycin ADR-to lipid ration. Oncol Rep. 14(5):1337-43.

Luce D, Bugel I, Goldberg P, Goldberg M, Salomon C, Billon-Galland M-A, Nicolau J, Quénel, Fevotte J, Brochard P. 2000. Environmental exposure to tremolite and respiratory cancer in New Calidonia: a case-control study. Am J Epidemiol. 151:259-65.

Lucesoli F, Fraga CG. 1995. Oxidative damage to lipids and DNA concurrent with decrease antioxidants in rat testes after acute iron intoxication. Arch Biochem Biophys. 31(6):5678-71.

——— 1999. Oxidative stress in testes of rats subjected to iron intoxication and alpha-tocopherol supplementation. Toxicology. 132(2):179-86.

Lucesoli G, Caligiuri M, Roberti MF, Perazzo JC, Frage CG. 1999. Dose-dependent increase of oxidative damage in the testes of rats subjected to acute iron overload. 372(1):37-43.

Lund EK, Fairweather-Tait SJ, Wharf SG, Johnson IT. 2001. Chronic exposure to high levels of dietary iron fortification increases lipid peroxidation in the mucosa of the rat large intestine. J Nutr. 131:2928-31.

Lund LG, Aust AE. 1990. Iron mobilization from asbestos by chelators and vitamin C. Arch Biochem Biophys. 278(1):61-4.

——— 1991a. Mobilization of iron from crocidolite asbestos by certain chelators results in enhanced crocidolite-dependent oxygen consumption. Arch Biochem Biophys. 287(1):91-6.

——— 1991b. Iron-catalysed reactions may be responsible for the biochemical and biological effects of asbestos. Biofactors 3:83-9.

——— 1992. Iron mobilization from crocidolite asbestos greatly enhances crocidolite-dependent formation of DNA single-strand breaks in X174 FRI DNA Carcinogenesis 13:637-42.

Lund LG, Williams MG, Dodson RF, Aust AE. 1994. Iron associated with asbestos bodies is responsible for the formation of single strand breaks in phi X174 RFI DNA. Occup Environ Med. 51(3):200-4.

MacDonald RA. 1964. Hemochromatosis and Hemosiderosis. Springfield, IL: Charles C Thomas Press.

Mader JS, Smyth D, Marshall J, Hoskin DW. 2006. Bovine lactoferricin inhibits basic fibroblast growth factor- and vascular endothelial growth factor 165-induced angiogenesis by competing for heparin-like binding sites on endothelial cells. Am J Pathol. 169(5):1753-66.

Maharaj DS, Maharaj H, Daya S, Glass BD. 2006. Melatonin and 6-hydroxymelatonin protect against iron-induced neurotoxicity. J Neurochem 96(1):78-81.

Mann VM, Cooper JM, Daniel SE, Srai K, Jenner P, Marsden CD, Schapira AH. 1995. Complex I, iron, and ferritin in Parkinson's disease substantia nigra. Ann Neurol. 36(6): 875-8.

Marcus DM, Zinberg N. 1975. Measurement of serum ferritin by radioimmunoassay: results in normal and individuals and patients with breast cancer. J Natl Cancer Inst. 55(4):791-5.

Masini A, Ceccarelli D, Giovannini F, Montosi G, Garuti C, Pietrangelo A. 2000. Iron-induced oxidant streas leads to irreversible mitochondrial dysfunctions and fibrosis in the liver of chronic iron-dosed gerbils. The effect of silybin. J Bioenerg Biomembr. 32(2):175-82.

McCord JM, Fridovich I. 1969. Superoxide dismutase: an enzymic function for erythroprein (hemocuprein). J Biol Chem. 244:6049.

McDonald JC, McDonald AD. 1996. The epidemiology of mesothelioma in historical context. Eur Respir J. 9:1932-1942.

Michaeli S, Oz G, Source DJ, Garwood M, Ugurbil K, Majestic S, Tuite P. 2007. Assessment of brain iron and neuronal integrity in patients with Parkinson's disease using novel MRI contrasts. Mov Disord. 22(3):334-40..

Millan, M, Sobrino T, Caswtellanos M, Nombela F, Arenillas JF, Riva E, Cristobo I, Garcìa MM, Vivancos J, Serena J, Morro MA, Castillo J, Dávalos A. 2007. Increased body iron stores are associated with poor outcome after thrombolytic treatment in acute stroke. Stroke. 38:90-5.

Mimura J, Fujii-Kuriyama Y. 2003. Functional role of AhR in the expression of toxic effects by TCDD. Biochim Biophys Acta. 1619(3):263-8.

Mistry N, Drobini P, Näslund J, Sunkari VG, Jenssen H, Evander M. 2007. Anti-papillomavirus activity of human and bovine lactoferrin. Antiviral Res. 75(3):258-65.

Miyasaki K, Murao S, Koizumi N. 1977. Hemochromatosis associated with brain lesions: a disorder of trace-metal binding proteins and/or polymers? J Neuropathol Exp Neurol. 36:664-76.

Mohan KV, Gunasedaran P, Varalakshmi E, Hara Y, Nagini S. 2007. In vitro evaluation of the anticancer effect of lactoferrin and tea polyphenol combination on oral carcinoma cells. Cell Biol Int. 31(6):599-608.

Mohan KV, Letchoumy PV, Hara Y, Nagini S. 2008. Combination chemoprevention of hamster buccal pouch carcinogenesis by bovine milk lactoferrin and black tea polyphenols. Cancer Invest. 26(2):193-201.

Montgomery EG Jr. 1995. Heavy metals and the etiology of Parkinson's disease and other movement disorders. Toxicology. 97(1-3):3-9.

Moore CA, Raha-Chowdhury R, Fagan DG, Worwood M. 1994. Liver iron concentrations in sudden infant death syndrome. 70($):295-8.

Moroz C, Kan M, Chaimof C, Marcus H, Kupfer B, Cuckle HS. 1984. Ferritin-bearing lymphocytes in the diagnosis of breast cancer. Cancer. 54(1):84-9.

Morris CM, Edwardson JA. 1994. Iron histochemistry of the substantia nigra in Parkinson's disease. Neurodegeneration. 3(4):277-82.

Mossman BT, Marsh JP, Shatos MA, Doherty J, Gilbert R, Hill S. 1987. Implication of active oxygen species as second messengers of asbestos toxicity. Drug Chem Toxicol. 10(1-2):157-80.

Mossman BT, Marsh JP, Shatos MA. 1986. Alteration of superoxide dismutase activity in tracheal epithelial cells by asbestos and inhibition of cytotoxicity by antioxidants. Lab Invest. 54(2):204-12.

Mossman BT, Marsh JP. 1989. Evidence supporting a role for active oxygen species in asbestos-induced toxicity and lung disease. Environ Health Perspect. 81:91-4.

Muir AR, Goldberg L. 1961. The tissue response to iron-dextran; an electron-microscope study. J Pathol Bacteriol. 82:471-82.

Murray MJ, Murray AB, Murray MB, Murray CJ. 1978. The adverse effect of iron repletion on the course of certain infections. Br Med J. 2:1113.

Nadarajah N, Van Hamme J, Pannu J, Singh A, Ward O. 2002. Enhanced transformation of polycyclic aromatic hydrocarbons using combined Eenton's reagent , microbial treatment and surfactants. Appl Microbiol Biotechnol. 59(4-5):540-4.

Nakano M. 1993. A possible mechanism of iron neurotoxicity. Eur Neurol. 33 Suppl:44-51.

Nakase I, Lai H, Singh NP, Sasaki T. 2007.Anticancer properties of artemisinin derivatives and their targeted delivery by trasferrin conjugation. Int J Pharm. [Epub ahead of print]

Nakase M, Inui M, Okumura K, Kamei T, Nakamura S, Tagawa T. 2005. p53 gene therapy of human osteosarcoma using a transferrin-modified cationic liposome. Mol Cancer Ther. 4(4):625-31.

Neilands JB. 1952. A crystalline organo-iron pigment from a rust fungus, *Ustilago sphaerogena.* 74:4846.

Nelson JM, Stevens RG. 1991. Ferritin-iron increases killing of Chinese hamster ovary cells by x irradiation. Cell Prolif. 24:411.

Nelson RL, Yoo SJ, Tanure JC, Andrianopoulos G, Misumi A. 1989. The effect of iron on experimental colorectal carcinogenesis. Anticancer Res. 9(6):1477-82.

Nelson RL. 2001. Iron and colorectal cancer risk: human studies. 2001. Iron and colorectal cancer risk: human studies. Nutr Rev. 59(5):140-8.

Nicholson WJ, Raffn E. 1995. Recent data on cancer due to asbestos in the U.S.A. and Denmark. Med Lav. 86(5):393-410.

Nielsen JE, Jensen LN, Drabbe K. 1995. Hereditary haemochromatosis: a case of iron accumulating in the basal ganglia associated with a parkinsonian syndrome. J Neurol Neurosurg Psychiatry. 59:318-21.

Nishina S, Hino K, Korenage M, Vecchi C, Pietrangelo A, Mizukami Y, Furutani T, Sakai A, Okuda M, Hidaka I, Okita K, Sakaida I. 2008. Hepatitis C virus-induced reactive oxygen species raise hepatic iron level in mice by reducing hepcidin transcription. Gastroenterology. 134(1):226-38.

Norat T, Bingham S, Ferrari P, Slimani N, Jenab M, Mazuir M, Overvod K, Olsen A, Tjønneland A, Clavel F, Boutron-Ruault M-C, Kesse E, Boeing H, Bergmann, MM, Nieters A, Linseisen J, Trichopoulou A, Trichopoulos D, Tountas Y, Berrino F, Palli D, Panico S, Tumino R, Vineis P, Bueno-de-Mesquita HB, Peeters PHM, Engeset D, Lund E, Skeie G, Ardanaz E, González C, Navarro C, Quirós JR, Sanchez M-J, Berglund G, Mattison I, Hallmans G, Palmqvist R, Day NE, Khaw K-T, Key TJ, San Joaquin M, Hémon B, Saracci R, Kaaks R, Riboli E. 2005. Meat, fish, and colorectal cancer risk: The European Prospective Investigation into Cancer and Nutrition. J Natl Cancer Inst. 97:906-16.

Norat T, Lukanova A, Ferrari P, Riboli E. 2002. Meat consumption and colorectal cancer risk: dose-responsive meta-analysis of epidemiological studies. Int J Cancer. 98(2):124-56.

Norat T, Riboli E. 2001. Meat consumption and colorectal cancer: a review of epidemiologic evidence. Nutr Rev. 59(2):37-47.

Oakley AE, Collingwood JF, Dobson J, Love G, Perrott HR, Edwardson JA, Elstner M, Morris CM. 2007. Individual dopaminergic neurons show raised iron levels in Parkinson disease. Neurology. 68:1820-25.

Oates PS, West AR. 2006. Heme in intestinal epithelial cell turnover, differentiation, detoxification, inflammation, carcinogenesis, absorption and motility. World J Gastroenterol. 12(27):4281-95.

Olanow CW, Marsden D, Perl D, Cohen G, eds. 1992. Iron and Oxidative Stress in Parkinson's Disease. Ann Neurol. 32:Suppl.

Olanow CW. 1992. An introduction to the free radical hypothesis in Parkinson's disease. Ann Neurol. 32 Suppl:S2-9.

Olynyk JK. 1999. Hepatitis C and iron. Keio J Med. 48(3):124-31.

Olynyk JK, Reddy KR, DiBisceglie AM, Jeffers LJ, Parker TI, Radick JL, Schiff ER, Fujisawa K, Marumo F, Sato C. 1995. Hepatic iron concentration as a predictor of response to interferon alpha therapy in chronic hepatitis C. Gastroenterology. 106(4):1104-9.

Ortega R, Cloetens P, Deves G, Carmona A, Bohics. 2007. Iron storage within dopamine neurovesicles revealed by chemical nano-imaging. PLoS ONE. 2(9)e925.

Owen AD, Schapira AH, Jenner P, Marsden CD. 1996. Oxidative stress and Parkinson's disease. Ann N Y Acad Sci. 12(1):73-94.

Owen RW, Spiegelhalder B, Bartsch H. 1998. Phytate, reactive oxygen species and colorectal cancer. Eur J Cancer Prev. 7 Suppl 2:S41-54.

Owen RW, Weisgerber UM, Spiegelhalder B, Bartsch H. 1996. Faecal phytic acid and its relation to other putative markers of risk for colorectal cancer. Gut. 38(4):591-7.

Owen RW, Weisgerber UM, Spiegelhalder B, Bartsch H. 1996. Faecal phytic acid and its relation other putative markers of risk of colorectal cancer. Gut. 38:591-7.

Ozdemir E, Dokucu AI, Uzunlar AK, Ece A, Yaldiz AK, Ece A, Yaldiz M, Oztürk H. 2002. Experimental study on effects of deferoxamine mesilate in emeliorating cisplatin-induced nephrotoxicity. Int Urol Nephrol. 33(1):127-31.

Papanastasiou DA, Vayenas DV, Vassilopoulos A, Repanti A. 2000. Concentration of iron and distribution of iron and transferrin after experimental iron overload in rat tissues in vivo: study of the liver, the spleen, the nervous system, and other organs. Pathol Res Pract. 196(1):47-54.

Papanikolaou G, Pantopoulos K. 2005. Iron metabolism and toxicity. Toxicology and Applied Pharmacology. 202:199-211.

Papenhausen PR, Emeson EE, Croft CB, Borowiecki B. 1984. Ferritin-bearing lymphocytes in patients with cancer. Cancer. 53(2):267-71.

Park CH, Valore EV, Waring AJ, Ganz T. 2001. Hepcidin, a urinary antimicrobial peptide synthesized in the liver. J Biol Chem. 278(11):7806-816.

Park SH, Aust AE. 1998a. Participation of iron and nitric oxide in the mutagenicity of asbestos in hgprt-, gpt+ Chinese hamster V79 cells. Cancer Res. 58(6):1144-8.

———— 1998b. Regulation of nitric oxide synthase induction by iron and glutathione in asbestos-treated human lung epithelial cells. Arch Biochem Biophys 360(1):47-52.

Pattanapanyasat K, Hoy TG, Jacobs A, Courtney S, Webster DF. 1988. Ferritin-bearing T-lymphocytes and serum ferritin in patients with breast cancer. Br J Cancer. 57(2):193-7.

Pereira MC, Pereira ML, Sousa JP. 1999. Histological effects of iron accumulation on mice liver and spleen after administration of a metallic solution. Biomaterials. 20(22):2193-8.

Perera D, Pizzey A, Campbell A, Katz M, Porter J, Petrou M, Irvine DS, Chatterjee R. 2002. Sperm DNA damage in potentially fertile homozygous ß-thalassaemia patients with iron overload. Human Reproduction. 17(7):1820-5.

Peterson DR. 2005. Alcohol, iron-associated oxidative stress, and cancer. Alcohol. 35(3):243-9.

Pierre F, Peiro G, Taché S, Cross AJ, Bingham NG, Gottardi G, Corpet DE, Guéraud F. 2006. New marker of colon cancer risk associated with heme intake: 1,4-dihydroxynonane mercapturic acid. Cancer Epidemiol

Biomarkers Prev. 15(11):2274-9.

Pietrangelo A. 2002. Mechanism of iron toxicity. Adv Exp Med Biol. 509:19-43.

——— 2003. Iron-induced oxidant stress in alcoholic liver fibrogenesis. Alcohol. 30(2):121-9.

Pigeon C, Turlin B, Iancu TC, Leroyer P, LeLan J, Deugnier Y, Brissot P, Loréal O. 1999. Carbonyl-iron supplementation induces hepatocyte nuclear changes in BALB/CJ male mice. J Hepatol. 30(5):926-34.

Pike MC, Spicer DV, Dahmoush L, Press MF. 1993. Estrogens, progestogens, normal breast cell proliferation, and breast cancer risk. Epidemiol Rev. 15:17-35.

Piperno A, Sampietro M, D'Alba R, Foffi L, Fargion S, Parma S, Nicoli C, Corbetta N, Pozzi M, Arosio V, Boari G, Fiorelli G. 1996. Iron stores, response to interferon therapy, and effect of iron depletion in chronic hepatitis C. Liver. 16(4):248-54.

Pippard MJ. 1994. *Secondary Iron Overload. London*: WB Saunders Company Ltd.

Porres JM, Stahl CC, Cheng WH, Fu Y, Roneker KR, Pond WG, Lei XG. 1999. Dietary intrinsic phytate protects colon from lipid peroxidation in pigs with a moderately high dietary iron intake. Proc Soc Exp Biol Med. 221(1):80-6.

Porter JB, Huens ER. 1989. The toxic effects of desferrioxamine. Balliere's Clin Haematol. 2:459-74.

Posey JE, Gherardini FC. 2000. Lack of a role for iron in the Lyme disease pathogen. Science. 288:1651.

Pouzard C, Tyrrell RM. 1999. Apoptosis, the role of oxidative stress and the example of solar UV rradiation. Photochem Photobiol. 70:380-90.

Pouzard C, Reelfs O, Kvam E, Tyrrell RM. 1999a. The iron regulatory protein can determine the effectiveness of 5-aminolevulinic acid in inducing protoporphyrin IX in human skin fibroblasts. J Invest Dermatol. 112:419-25.

Pouzard C, Watkin RD, Brown JE, Tyrrell. 1999b. Ultraviolet radiation induces immediate release of iron in human primary skin fibroblasts: The role of ferritin. Proc Natl Acad Sci USA. 96:6751-6.

Prieto J, Barry M, Sherlock S. 1975. Serum ferritin in patients with iron overload and with acute and chronic liver diseases. Gastroenterology. 68:525-33.

Prutki M, Poljak-Blazi M, Jakopovic M, Tomas D, Stipanci I, Zarkovic N. 2006. Altered iron metabolism, transferrin receptor 1 and ferritin in patients with colon cancer. Cancer Lett. 238(2):188-96.

Pun SH, Tack, F, Bellocq NC, Cheng J, Grubbs BH, Jensen GS, Davis ME, Brewster M, Janicot M, Janssens B, Floren W, Bakker A. 2004. Targeted delivery of RNA-cleaving DNA Enzyme (DNAzyme) to tumor tissue by transferrin-mocified, cyclodextrin-based particles. Cancer Biol and Ther. 3:7641-50.

Purohit V, Russo D, Salin M. 2003. Role of iron in alcoholic liver disease: introduction and summary of the symposium. Alcohol. 30(2):93-7.

Raha-Chowhury R, Moore CA, Bradley D, Henley R, Worwood M. 1996. Blood ferritin concentrations in newborns and the sudden infant death syndrome. J Clin Pathol. 49:168-70.

Raje D, Mukhtar H, Oshowo A, Ingham Clark C. 2007. What proportion of patients referred to secondary care with iron deficiency anemia have colon cancer: Dis Colon Rectum. 50(8):1211-4.

Rajesh Kumar T, Doreswamy K, Shrilatha B, Muralidhra. 2002. Oxidative stress associated DNA damage in testis of mice: induction of abnormal sperms and effects on fertility. Mutat Res. 513(1,2):103-11.

Rakba N, Loyer P, Gilot D, Delcros JG, Glaise D, Baret PPierre JL, Brissot P, Lescoat G. 2000. Antiproliferative and apoptotic effects of O-Trensox, a new synthetic iron chelator, on differentiated hepatoma cell lines. Carcinogenesis. 21:943-51.

Randerath E, Danna TF, Randernath K. 1992. DNA damage induced by cigarette smoke condensate in vitro as assayed by 32P-postlabeling. Comparison with cigarette smoke-associated DNA adduct profiles in vivo.

Reelfs O, Tyrrell RM, Pourzand C. 2004. Ultraviolet A radiation-immediate iron release is a key modulator of the activation of NF-$_\kappa$B in human skin fibroblasts. 122:1440-7.

Reizenstein P. 1991. Iron, free radicals and cancer. Med Oncol Tumor Pharmacother. 8(4):229-33.

Repine JE, Pfenninger OW. Talmage DW, Berger EM, Pettijohn DE. 1981. Dimethylsulfoxide prevents DNA nicking mediated by ionizing radiation or iron/hydrogen peroxide generated gydroxyl radical. Proc Natl Acad Sci. 78:1001.

Report on Carcinogens. 2002. Iron Dextran Complex. Reasonably anticipated to be a human carcinogen. First listed in the Second Annual Report on Carcinogens (1981).

Rezazadeh H, Athar M. 1997. Evidence that iron-overload promotes 7,12-dimethylbenz(a)anthracene-induced skin tumorigenesis in mice. Redox Rep. 3(5-6):303-9.

Richmond HG. 1959. Induction of sarcoma in the rat by iron-dextran complex. Br Med J. 1(5127):947-49.

————— 1960a. The carcinogenicity of an iron-dextran complex. J Natl Cancer Inst. 24:109-47.

————— 1960b. The carcinogenicity of an iron-dextran complex. Cancer Prog. 1960:24-33.

Riederer P, Lange KW. 1992. Pathogenesis of Parkinson's disease. Curr Opin Neurol Neurosurg. 5(3):1080-9.

Riederer P, Sofic E, Rausch WD, Schmidt B, Reynolds GP, Jellinger K, Youdim MB. 1989. Transition metals, ferritin, glutathione, and ascorbic acid in parkinsonian brains. J Neurochem. 52(2):515-20.

Rimbach G, Pallauf J. 1998. Phytic acid inhibits free radical formation in vitro but does not affect liver oxidant or antioxidant status in growing rats. J Nutr. 128(11):1950-5.

Robinson CE, Bell DN, Sturdy JH. 1960. Possible association of malignant neoplasm with iron-dextran injection. A case report. Br Med J. 2(5199):648-50.

Rocchi E, Gibertini P, Cassanelli M, Pietrangelo A, Borghi A, Ventura E. 1986. Serum ferritin in the assessment of liver iron overload and iron removal therapy in porphyria cutanea tarda. Lab Clin Med. 107(1):36-42.

Roe FJ, Carter RL. 1967. Iron-dextran carcinogenesis in rats: influence of dose on the number and types of neoplasm induced. Int J Cancer. 2(4):370-80.

Roe FJ, Haddow A, Dukes CE, Mitchley BC. 1964. Iron-dextran carcinogenesis in rats: effect of distributing injected material between one, two, four, or six sites. Br J Cancer. 18:801-8.

Roe FJ, Lancester MC. 1964. Natural, metallic and other substances as carcinogens. Br Med Bull. 20:127-33.

Rojas G, Messen L. 1968. Generalized cytosiderosis in two cases of progressive myoclonic epilepsy with Lafora inclusion bodies. Histopathological and ultrastructural studies. Neurocirugia. 26:3-11.

Rosen HR, Moroz C, Reiner A, Reinerova M, Stierer M, Svec J, Schemper M, Jakesz R. 1992a. Placental isoferritin associated p43 antigen correlates with reatures of high differentiation in breast cancer. Breast Cancer Res Treat. 24(1):17-26.

————— 1992b. Expression of p43 in breast cancer tissue, correlation with prognostic parameters. Cancer Lett. 67(1):35-45.

Rosen HR, Stierer M, Göttlicher J, Wolf H, Weber R, Vogl E, Eibi M. 1992c. Determination of placental ferritin (PLF)-positive lymphocytes in women in early stages of breast cancer. Int J Cancer. 52(2):229-33.

Rouault TA, Cooperman S. 2006. Brain iron metabolism. Semin Pediatr Neurol. 13(3):142-8.

Rouault TA. 2003. Hepatic iron overload in alcoholic liver disease: why does it occur and what is its role in pathogenesis? Alcohol. 30(2):103-6.

Sadava D, Phillips T. Lin C, Kane SE. 2002. Transferrin overcomes drug resistance to artemisinin in human small-cell lung carcinoma cells. Cancer Lett. 179(2):151-6.

Saffiotti U, Montesano R, Sellakumar AR, Cefis F, Kaufman DG. 1972. Respiratory tract carcinogenesis induced by different numbers of administrations of benza(á)pyrene and ferric oxide. Cancer Res. 32:1073-81.

Sahoo SK, Labhasetwar V. 2005. Enhanced antiproliferative activity of transferrin-conjugated pacilitaxel-loaded nanoparticles is mediated via sustained intracellular drug retention. Mol Pharm. 2(5):373-83.

Sahu SC, Washington MC. 1991. Iron-mediated oxidative DNA damage detected by fluorometric analysis of DNA unwinding in isolated rat liver nuclei. Biomed Environ Sci. 4(3):219-28.

Salazar J, Mena N, Nunez MT. 2006. Iron dyshomeostasis in Parkinson's disease. J Neural Transm Suppl. 71:205-13.

Sampietro M, Fiorelli G, Fargion S. 1999. Iron overload in porphyria cutanea tarda. Haematologica. 84:248-53.

Santangelo C, Vari R, Seazzocchio B, De Benedetto R, Filesi C, Masella R. 2007. Polyphenols, intracellular signaling and inflammation. Ann Ist Super Sanita. 43(4):394-405.

Sardi B. 1999. *The Iron Time Bomb*. San Dimas, CA: Bill Sardi.

Sawa T, Akaike T, Kida K, Fukushima Y, Koichi T, Maeda H. 1998. Lipid peroxyl radicals from oxidized oils and heme-iron: implications of a high-fat diet in colon carcinogenesis. Cancer Epidemiol Biomarkers Prev. 7:1007-12.

Schulman I. 1960. Experimental carcinogenesis with iron-dextran. Pediatrics. 26:347-50.

Schümann K, Borch-Iohnsen B, Hentze MW, Marx JJM. 2002. Tolerable upper intakes for dietary iron set by the US Food and Nutrition Board. Am J Clin Nutr. 76:49-500.

Séité S, Popovic E, Verdier MP, Roguet R, Portes P, Cohen C, Fourtanier A, Galey JB.. 2004. Iron chelation can modulate UVA-induced lipid peroxidation and ferritin expression in human reconstructed epidermis. Photodermatol Photoimmunol Photochem. 20:47-52.

Seitz HK, Stickel R. 2006. Risk factors and mechanisms of hepato-carcinogenesis with special emphasis on alcohol and oxidative stress. Biol Chem. 387(4):349-60.

Selby JV, Friedmann GD. 1988. Epidemiological evidence of an association of body iron stores and risk of cancer. Int J Cancer. 41:677.

Selim MH, Ratan RR. 2004. The role of iron neurotoxicity in ischemic stroke. 2004. Ageing Res Rev. 3(3):345-53.

Senesse P, Meance S, Cottet V, Faivre J, Boutron-Ruault MC. 2004. High dietary iron and copper: a case control study in Burgundy, France. Nutr Cancer. 49(1):66-71.

Sengstock GJ, Olanow CW, Dunn AJ, Arendash GW. 1992. Iron induces degeneration of nigrostriatal neurons. Brain Res Bull. 28(4):645-9.

Seril DN, Liao J, Yang GY, Yang CS. 2003. Oxidative stress and ulcerative colitis-associated carcinogenesis: studies in humans and animal models. Carcinogenesis. 24(3):353-62.

Sesnik ALA, Termont DSML, Kleibeuker JH, Van der Meer R. 1999. Red meat and colon cancer: the cytotoxic and hyperproliferative effects of dietary heme. 1999. Cancer Res. 59:5704-9.

Shade AL, Caroline L. 1944. Raw hen egg white and the role of iron in growth inhibition of *Shigella dysenteria, Staphylococcus aureus, Escherichia coli, and Saccharomyces cerevisiae.* Science. 100:14-15.

——— 1946. An iron-binding component in human blood plasma. Science. 104:340-41.

Shan Y, Lambrecht RW, Bonkovsky HL. 2005. Association of hepatitis C virus infection with serum iron status: analysis of data from the third National Health and Nutrition Examination Survey. Clin Infect Dis. 40(6):834-41.

Sharma JB, Jain S, Mallika V, et al. 2004. A prospective, partially randomized study of pregnancy outcomes and hematologic responses to oral and intramuscular iron treatment in moderately anemic pregnant women. Am J Clin Nutr. 79:116-22.

Shatos MA, Doherty JM, Marsh JP, Mossman BT. 1987. Prevention of asbestos-induced cell death in rat lung fibroblasts and alveolar macrophages by scavengers of active oxygen species. Environ Res. 44(1):103-16.

Sheldon JH. 1935. Haemochromatosis. Oxford Univ Press, London.

Shen HM, Ong CN, Shi CY. 1995. Involvement of reactive oxygen species in aflatoxin B1-induced cell injury in cultured rat hepatocytes. Toxicology. 99(1-2):115-23.

Shen Z, Bosbach D, Hochella MF Jr, Bish DL, Williams MG Jr, Dodson RF, Aust AE. 2000. Using in vitro iron deposition on asbestos to model asbestos bodies formed in human lung. Chem Res Toxicol. 13(9):913-21.

Shimamura M, Yamamoto Y, Ashino H, Oikawa T, Hazato T, Tsuda H, Iigo M. 2004. Bovine lactoferrin inhibits tumor-induced angiogenesis. Int J Cancer. 111(1):111-6.

Shimida T, Fujji-Kuriyama T. 2004. Metabolic activation of polycyclic aromatic hydrocarbons to carcinogens by cytochromes P450 1A1 and 1B1. Cancer Sci. 95:1-6.

Shimida T. 2006. Xenobiotic-metabolizing enzymes involved in activation and detoxification of carcinogenic polycyclic aromatic hydrocarbons. Drug Metab Pharmacokinet. 21(4):257-76.

Shoham S, Youdim MB. 2004. Nutritional iron deprivation attenuates kainite-induced neurotoxicity in rats: implications for involvement of iron in neurodegeneration. Ann N Y Acad Sci. 1012:94-114.

Shterman N, Kupfer B, Moroz C. 1991. Comparison of transferrin receptors, iron content and isoferritin profile in normal and malignant human breast cell lines. Pathobiology. 59(1):19-25.

Simonart T, Boelaert JR, Andrei G, van den Oord JJ, Degraef C, Hermans P, Noel JC, Van Vooren JP, Heenen M, De Clercq E, Snoeck R. 2002. Desferrioxamine enhances AISA-associated Kaposi's sarcoma tumor development in a xenograft model. Int J Cancer. 100:140-3.

Singh S, Khodr H, Taylor M, Hider RC. 1995. Therapeutic iron chelators and their potential side-effects. Biochem Soc Symp. 61:127-37.

Smith KR, Aust AE. 1997. Mobilization of iron from urban particulates leads to generation of reactive oxygen species in vitro and induction of ferritin synthesis in human lung epithelial cells. Chem Res Toxicol. 10(7):828-34.

Smith KR, Vernath JM, Hu AA, Lighty JS, Aust AE. 2000. Interleukin-8 levels in human lung epithelial cells are increased in response to coal fly ash and vary with bioavailability of iron, as a function of particle size and source of coal. Chem Res Toxicol. 13(2):118-25.

Smith Sl, Maggs JL, Edwards G, Ward SA, Park BK, McLean WG. 1998. The role of iron in neurotoxicity: a study of novel antimalarial drugs. Neurotoxicity. 19(4-5):557-9.

Sofic E, Paulus W, Jellinger K, Riederer P, Youdim MB. 1991. Selective increase of iron in substantia nigra zona compacta of parkinsonian brains. J Neurochem. 56(3):978-82.

Sofic E, Riederer P, Heinsen H, Beckmann H, Reynolds GP, Hebenstreit G, Youdim MB. 1988. Increased iron (III) and total iron content in post mortem substantia nigra of parkinsonian brain. J Neural Transm. 74:199-205.

Solomons NW, Schümann K. 2004. Intramuscular administration of iron dextran is inappropriate for treatment of moderate pregnancy anemia, both in intervention research on underprivileged women and in routine prenatal care provided by public health services. Am J Clin Nutr. 79(1):1-3.

Song BB, Anderson DJ, Schacht J. 1997. Protection from gentamicin ototoxicity by iron chelators in guinea pig *in vivo*. J Pharmacol Exp Therap. 282:369-77.

Song BB, Sha SH, Schacht J. 1998. Iron chelators protect from aminoglycoside-induced cochleo- and vestibulo-toxicity. Free Radic Biol Med. 25(2):189-95.

Stål P, Johansson I, Ingelman-Sundberg M, Hagen K, Hultcrantz R. 1996. Hepatotoxicity induced by iron overload and alcohol. Studies on the role of chelatable iron, cytochromes P450 2E1 and lipid peroxidation. J Hepatol. 25(4)"538-46.

Stål P. 1995. Iron as a hepatotoxin. Dig Dis. 13(4):205-22.

Stankiewicz J, Panter SS, Neema M, Arora A, Batt CE, Bakshi R. 2007. Iron in chronic brain disorders: imaging and neurotherapeutic implications. Neurotherapeutics. 4(3):37-86.

Stevens RG, Beasley RP, Blumberg BS. 1986. Iron-binding proteins and risk of cancer in Taiwan. J Natl Cancer Inst. 76(4):605-10.

Stevens RG, Graubard BI, Micozzi MS, Neriishi K, Blumberg BS. 1994. Moderate elevation of body iron level and increased risk of cancer occurrence and death. Int J Cancer. 56(3)364-9.

Stevens RG, Jones DY, Micozzi MS, Taylor PR. 1988. Body iron stores and the risk of cancer. N Engl J Med.319:1047-52.

Stevens RG, Kalkwarf DR. 1990. Iron, radiation, and cancer. Env Health Persp. 87:291-300.

Stevens RG, Morris JE, Anderson LE. 2000. Hemochromatosis heterozygotes may constitute a radiation-sensitive subpopulation. Radiat Res. 153(6):844-7.

Stevens RG. 1990. Iron and the risk of cancer. Med Oncol Tumor Pharmacother. 7(2-3):177-81.

——— 1991. Dietary effects on breast cancer. Lancet. 338(8760):186-7.

——— 1992. Iron and cancer. In: *Iron and Human Disease.* Lauffer RB, ed. Boca Raton, Ann Arbor, London, Tokyo: CRC Press, pp 333-47.

Stone WL, Papas AM, LeClair IO, Qui M, Ponder T. 2002. The influence of dietary iron and tocopherols on oxidative stress and ras-p21 levels in the colon. Cancer Detect Prev. 26(1):78-84.

Strachan AS. 1929. MD Thesis. University of Glasgow.

Sullivan JL. 1981. Iron and the sex differences in heart disease risk. Lancet. 1(8233):1293-4.

——— Stored iron as a risk factor for ischemic heart disease. In: Lauffer RB, ed. *Iron and Human Disease.* Boca Raton, Ann Arbor, London, Tokyo: CRC Press, 1992.

Sulzer D, Schmitz Y. 2007. Parkinson's disease: return of an old prime suspect. Neuron. 55:8-10.

Sumida Y, Kanemasa K, Fukumoto K, Yoshida N, Sakai K. 2007. Effects of dietary iron reduction versus phlebotomy in patients with chronic hepatitis C: results from a randomized, controlled trial on 40 Japanese patients. Intern Med. 46(10):637-42.

Sun-Hee P, Aust AE. 1998. Participation of iron and nitric oxide in mutagenicity of asbestos in hgprt-, gpt+ Chinese hamster V79 cells. Cancer Res. 58:1144-48.

Sutnik AJ, Blumberg BS, Lustbader ED. 1974. Elevated serum iron levels and persistent Australian antigen (HBsAg). Ann Intern Med. 81:855-6.

Suzuki Y, Saito H, Suzuki M, Hosoki Y, Sakurai S, Fujimoto Y, Kohgo Y. 2002. Up-regulation of transferrin receptor expression in hepatocytes by habitual alcohol drinking is implicated in hepatic iron overload in alcoholic liver disease. Alcohol Clin Exp Res. 26(8 Suppl): 265-315.

Swaiman KF. 1991. Hallervorden-Spatz syndrome and brain iron metabolism. Arch Neurol. 48:1285-93.

Swaminathan S, Shah SV. 2008. Novel approaches targeted toward oxidative stress for the treatment of chronic kidney disease. Curr Opin Nephrol Hypertens. 17(2):143-8.

Swanson CA. 2003. Iron intake and regulation: implications for iron deficiency and iron overload. Alcohol. 30(2):99-102.

Takanashi M, Mochizuki H, Yokomizo K, Hattori N, Mori H, Yamamura Y, Mizuno Y. 2001. Iron accumulation in the substantia nigra of autosomal recessive juvenile parkinsonism (ARJJP). Parkinsonism Relat Disord. 7(4):311-13.

Talley NJ, Chute CG, Larson DE, Epstein R, Lydick EG, Melton LJ 3rd. 1989. Risk for colorectal adenocarcinoma in pernicious anemia. A population-based cohort study. Ann Intern Med. 111(9):738-42.

Tanaka M, Sotomatsu A, Kanai H, Hirai S. 1991. Dopa and dopamine caused cultured neuronal death in the presence of iron. J Neurol Sci. 101(2):198-203.

Tappel A. 2007. Heme of consumed red meat can act as a catalyst of oxidative damage and could initiate colon, breast and prostate cancers, heart disease and other diseases. Med Hypothesis. 68(3):562-4.

Temlett JA, Landsberg JP, Watt F, Grime GW. 1994. Increased iron in the substantis nigra compacta of the MPTP-lesioned hemiparkinsonian African green monkey: evidence from proton microprobe elemental microanalysis. J Neurochem. 62(1):134-46.

Tepel M. 2007. N-acetylcysteine in the prevention of ototoxicity. Kidney Int. 72(3):231-2.

Terada LS, Willingham IR, Repine JE. 1992. Iron and stroke. In: *Iron and Human Disease.* Boca Raton, Ann Arbor, London, Tokyo: CRC Press, pp 313-332.

Thedering F. 1964. The tolerance of iron therapy with special reference to the carcinogenic effect of the dextran-iron complex. Med Welt. 17:277-82.

Thompson CM, Marksberry WR, Ehmann WD, Mao YY, Vance DE. 1988. Regional brain trace-element studies in Alzheimer's disease. Neurotoxicology. 9:1.

Todorich BM, Connor JR. 2004. Redox metals in Alzheimer's disease. Ann NY Acad Sci. 1012:171-78.

Topham RW, Walker MC, Callisch MP, Williams RW. 1982. Evidence for the participation of intestinal xanthine oxidase in the mucosal processing of iron. Biochemistry. 21:4529.

Trobini P, Mauri V, Salvioni A, Corengia C, Arosio C, Piperno A. 2001. S65C frequency in Italian patients with hemochromatosis, porphyria cutanea tarda and viral hepatitis with iron overload. Hematologica. 86:316-7.

Trousseau A. 1865. Clinique Méd de l'Hôtel de Paris (2d edit). 2:663-98.

Tsuda H, Sekine K, Fujita K, Ligo M. 2002. Cancer prevention by bovine lactoferrin and underlying mechanisms – a review of experimental and clinical studies. Biochem Cell Biol. 80(1):131-6.

Tsuda H, Sekine K, Ushida Y, Kuhara T, Takasuka N, Iigo M, Han BS, Moore MA. 2000. Milk and dairy products in cancer prevention: focus on bovine lactoferrin. Mutat Res. 462(2-3):227-33.

Tsuda H, Sekine K. 2000. Milk components as cancer chemopreventive agents. Asian Pac J Cancer Prev. 1(4):277-82.

Turlin B, Deugnier Y. 2002. Iron overload disorders. Clin Liver Dis. 6(2):481-96.

Turner HM, Grace HG. 1938. An investigation into cancer mortality among males in certain Sheffield trades. J Hyg 38:90-103.

Turver CJ, Brown RC. 1987. The role of catalytic iron in asbestos induced lipid peroxidation and DNA-strand breakage in C3H10T1/2 cells. Br J Cancer. 56(2):133-6.

Tyrrell RM. 1991. UVA (320-380 nm) radiation as an oxidative stress. In: Sies H, ed. *Oxidative Stress: Oxidants and Antioxidants*. London: Academic Press, pp 57-83.

——— 1996. Activation of mammalian gene expression by the UV component of sunlight – from models to reality. Bioassays. 18:139-48.

Ulbrich EJ, Lebrecht A, Schneider I, Ludwig E, Koelbl H, Hefler LA. 2003. Serum parameters of iron metabolism in patients with breast cancer. Anticancer Res. 23(6D):5107-9.

Valenti L, Pulixi EA, Arosio P, Cremonesi L, Biasiotto G, Dongiovanni P, Maggioni M, Fargion S, Fracanzani AL. 2007. Relative contribution of iron genes, dysmetabolism and hepatitis C virus (HCV)in the pathogenesis of altered iron regulation in HCV chronic hepatitis. Haematologica 92(8):1037-42.

Valk J. 1989. Magnetic Resonance of Myelin, Myelination and Myelin Disorders. New York: Springer-Verlag.

Valko M, Morris H, Mazúr M, Rapta P, Bilton RF. 2001. Oxygen free radical generating mechanisms in the colon: do the semiquinones of vitamin K play a role in the aetology of colon cancer? Biochim Biophys Acta. 1527(3):161-6.

Valko M, Rhodes CJ, Moncol J, Izakovic M, Mazur M. 2006. Free radicals, metals and antioxidants in oxidative stress-induced cancer. Chem Biol Interact. 160(1):1-40.

Vallier J, Rebouillat M. 1962. [Research on the in vivo carcinogenic activity of an iron-dextran complex in the rat.] CR Seances Soc Biol Fil. 156:691-93. (French)

van der A DL, Grobbee DE, Roest M, Mars JJ, Voorbij HA, van der Schouw YT. Serum ferritin is a risk factor for stroke in postmenopausal. 36(8):1637-41.

van Maanen JM, Borm Pj, Knaapen A, van Herwijnen M, Schilderman PA, Smith KR, Aust AE, Tomatis M, Fubini B. 1999. In vitro effects of coal fly ashes: hydroxyl radical generation, iron release, and DNA damage and toxicity in rat lung epithelial cells. Inhal Toxicol. 11(12):1123-41.

Van Thiel DH, Friedlander L, Faginoli S, Wright HI, Irish W, Gavaler JS. 1994. Response to interferon á therapy is influenced by the iron content of the liver. J Hepatol. 20:410-5.

Vandewalle B, Granier AM, Peyrat JP, Bonneterre J, Lefebvre J. 1985. Transferrin receptors in cultured breast cancer cells. J Cancer Res Clin Oncol. 110(1):71-6.

Varadhachary A, Wolf JS, Petrak K, O'Malley BW Jr, Spadaro M, Curcio C, Forni G, Pericle F.2004. Oral lactoferrin results in T cell-dependent tumor inhibition of head and neck squamous cell carcinoma in vivo. Int J Cancer. 111(3):398-403.

Vayanes DV, Repanti M, Vassilopoulor A, Papenstasiou DA. 1998. Influence ofiron overload on magnesium, zinc, and copper concentration in rat tissues in vivo. Study of liver, spleen, and brain. Int J Clin Lab Res. 28(3):183-6.

Vecchiola A, Asenjo A, Varleta J, Weinstein V, Oberhauser I. 1966. [Iron in the blood, cerebrospinal fluid and urine in patients with Parkinson's disease and in patients without this disorder (primary report).] Neurocirugia. 24(3):129-30. [Text in Spanish.]

Vile GF, Tanew-Ilitschew A, Tyrell RM. 1995. Activation of NF-kappa B in human skin fibroblasts by the oxidative stress generated by UVA radiation. Photochem Photobiol. 62:463-8.

Vile GF, Tyrrell RM. 1995. UVA radiation-induced oxidative damage to lipids and proteins in vitro and in human skin fibroblasts is dependent on iron and singlet oxygen. Free Radic Biol Med. 18:721-30.

Vogiatzi MG, Autio KA, Schneider R, Giardina PJ. 2004. Low bone mass in prepubertal children with Thalassemia major: insights into the pathogenesis of low bone mass in Thalassemia. J Ped Endocrinol & Metab. 17:1415-21.

Vrbanec D, Petriceviæ B. 2007. Estrogen and progesterone receptor status in primary breast cancer – a study of 11,273 patients from the year 1990-2002. Coll Antropol. 31(2):535-40.

Walker ARP, Arvidsson UB. 1953. Iron 'overload' in South African Bantu. J R Soc Trop Med Hyg. 47:536-48.

Ward PP, Paz E, Conneely OM. 2005. Multifunctional roles of lactoferrin: a critical overview. Cell Mol Life Sci. 62(22):2540-8.

Warder, M. 1984. *The Bronze Killer. Hemochromatosis: The No. 1 Genetic Disorder*. Delta, BC, Canada: Imperani Publishers.

Warheit DB, Hill LH, Brody AR. 1984. In vitro effects of crocidolite asbestos and wollastonite on pulmonary macrophages and serum complement. Scan Electron Microsc. (Pt 2):919-26.

Weinberg ED. 1966. Roles of metallic ions in host-parasite interactions. Bact Reviews. 30:1336-51.

———— 1974. Iron and susceptibility to infectious disease. Science. 184:952-56.

———— 1981. Iron and neoplasia. Biol Trace Elem Res. 3:55-80.

———— 1984. Iron withholding: a defence against infection and neoplasia. Physiol Rev. 64:65-102.

———— 1989. Iron, asbestos, and carcinogenicity. Lancet. 1:1399-40.

———— 1992a. Roles of iron in neoplasia: promotion, prevention and therapy. Biol Trace Elem Res. 34:123-40.

———— 1992b. Iron depletion: a defence against intracellular infection and neoplasia. Life Sci. 50:1289-97.

———— 1993. Association of iron with respiratory tract neoplasia. J Trace Elem Exp Med. 6:117-23.

———— 1994. Role of iron in colorectal cancer. BioMetals. 7:211-6.

———— 1996. Iron withholding: a defense against viral infections. BioMetals. 9:393-9.

———— 1996a. The role of iron in cancer. Euro J Cancer Prev. 5:19-36.

———— 2001. Elevated iron, antibiotics and hearing loss. Iron Disorders Institute. 2nd Quarter 2001, p 9.

———— 2001. Lung cancer among industrial sand workers exposed to crystalline silica. Am J Epidemiology. 154(3):288.

———— 2002. Therapeutic potential of human transferrin and lactoferrin. ASM News. 68(2):65-69.

———— 2004. *Exposing the Hidden Dangers of Iron*. Nashville, TN: Cumberland House.

———— 2005. Iron withholding as a defense strategy. In: Weiss G, Gordeuk VR, Hershko C, eds. *Anemia of Chronic Disease*. Boca Raton: Taylor & Francis.

———— 2006. Iron loading: a risk factor for osteoporosis. BioMetals. 19:633-35.

———— 2007. Antibiotic properties and applications of lactoferrin. Cur Pharm Design. 13:801-811.

Weinstein RE, Bond BH, Silberberg BK, Vaughn CB, Subbaiah P, Pieper DR. 1989. Tissue ferritin concentration and prognosis in carcinoma of the breast. Breast Cancer Res Treat. 14(3):349-53.

Weintraub LR, Edwards CQ, Krikker M. 1988. Hemochromatosis. Proceedings of the First International Conference. Ann NY Acad Sci. Volume 256.

Weiss G, Gordeuk VR, Hershko, eds. 2005. *Anemia of Chronic Disease*. Boca Raton: FL: Taylor and Francis.

Weitzman SA, Graceffa P. 1984. Asbestos catalyzes hydroxyl and superoxide radical generation from hydrogen peroxide. Arch Biochem Biophys. 228(1):373-6.

Weizer-Stern O, Adamsky K, Margalit O, Ashur-Favian O, Givol D, Amariglio N, Rechavi G. 2007. Hepcidin, a key regulator of iron metabolism, is transcriptionally activated by p53. Br J Haematol. 138(2):253-62.

Wellejus A, Poulsen HD, Loft S. 2000. Iron-induced oxidative DNA damage in rat sperm cells in vivo and in vitro. Free Radic Res. 32(1):75-83.

Wersinger C, Sidhu A. 2006. An inflammatory pathomechanism for Parkinson's disease? Curr Med Chem. 13(5):591-602.

Whiting RF, Wei L, Stitch HF. 1981. Chromosome-damaging activity of ferritin and its relation to chelation and reduction of iron. Cancer Res. 41:1628.

Whittaker P, Dunkel VC, Bucci TJ, Kusewitt DF, Thurman JD, Warbritton A, Wolff GL. 1997. Genome-linked toxic responses to dietary iron overload. Toxicol Pathol. 25(6):556-64.

Whittaker P, Dunkel VC, Seifried HE, Clarke JJ, San RHC. 2002. Evaluation of iron chelators for assessing the mechanism of genotoxicity of iron compounds. FDA Science Forum Poster Abstract, Board Z-06.

Whittaker P, Hines FA, Robl MG, Dunkel VC. 1996. Histopathological evaluation of liver, pancreas, spleen, and heart from iron-overloaded Sprague-Dawley rats. Toxicol Path. 24(5):558-63.

Whittaker P, Tufaro PR, Dunkel VC, Rader JI. 2001. Fortification of Iron and Folate in Cereals. FDA Science Forum Poster Abstract, Board P02.

Whitton, PS. 2007. Inflammation as a causative factor in the aetiology of Parkinson's disease. Br J Pharmacol. 150(8):963-76.

Witte DL, Crosby WH, Edwards CO, Fairbanks VF, Mitros FA. 1996. Practice guideline development task force of the College of American Pathologists: hereditary hemochromatosis. Clin Chim Acta. 245:139-200.

Wolf JS, Li G, Varadhachary A, Petrak K, Schneyer M, Li D, Ongkaesuwan M, Zhang X, Taylor RJ, Strome SE, O'Makket BW Jr. 2007. Oral lactoferrin results in T cell-dependent tumor inhibition of head and neck squamous cell carcinoma in vivo. Clin Cancer Res. 13(5);1601-10.

Wong RW, Richa DC, Hahn P, Green WR, Dunaief JL. 2007. Iron toxicity as a potential factor in AMD. Retina. 27:997-1003.

Wright A, Donaldson K, Davis JM. 1983. Cytotoxic effect of asbestos on macrophages in different activation states. 51:109-17.

Wright RO, Baccarelli A. 2007. Metals and neurotoxicology. J Nutr. 137(12):2809-13.

Wurzelmann JI, Silver A, Schreinemachers DM, Sandler RS, Everson RB. 1996. Iron intake and the risk of colorectal cancer. Cancer Epidemiol Biomarkers and Prev. 5:503-7.

Wyllie S, Liehr JG. 1997. Release of iron from ferritin storage by redox cycling of stilbene and steroid estrogen metabolites: a mechanism of induction of free radical damage by estrogen. Arch Biochem Biophys. 346(2):180-6.

Xiong S, She H, Sung CK, Tsukamoto H. 2003. Iron-dependent activation of NF-kappaB in Kuppfer cells: a priming mechanism for alcoholic liver disease. Alcohol. 30(2):107-13.

Xu A, Wu LJ, Santella RM, Hei TK. 1999. Role of oxyradicals in mutagenicity and DNA damage induced by crocidolite asbestos in mammalian cells. Cancer Res. 59(23):5922-6.

Xu A, Zhou H, Yu DZ, Hei TK. 2002. Mechanisms of the genotoxicity of crocidolite asbestos in mammalian cells: implication from mutation patterns by reactive oxygen species. Environ Health Perspect. 110(10):1003-8.

Xudong H, Moir RD, Tanzi RE, Bush AL, Rogers JT. 2004. Redox-active metals, oxidative stress, and Alzheimer's disease pathology. Ann NY Acad Sci. 1012:153-63.

Xue W, Warshawsky D. 2005. Metabolic activation of polycyclic and heterocyclic aromatic hydrocarbons and DNA damage: a review. Toxicol Appl Pharmacol. 206(1):73-93.

Yamasoba T, Schacht J, Shoji F, Miller JM. 1999. Attenuation of chochlear damage from nois trauma by an iron chelator, a free radical scavenger and glial cell-line-derived neutrotrophic factor in vivo. Brain Res. 815(2):317-25.

Yamauchi K, Wakabayashi H, Shin K, Takase M. 2006. Bovine lactoferrin: benefits and mechanisms of action against infections. Biochem Cell Biol. 84(3):291-6.

Yantin F, Andersen JK. 1999. The role of iron in Parkinson disease and 1-methyl-4-phenyl-1,2,3,6-tehydropyridine toxicity. IUBMB Life.

48(2):139-41.

Yiakouvaki A, Savovic J, Al-Quenaei A, Dowden J, Pourzand C. 2006. Caged-iron chelators a novel approach towards protecting skin cells against UVA-induced necrotic cell death. J Invest Dermatol. 126:2287-95.

Yoo MS, Chun HS, Son JJ, DiGiorgio LA, Kim DJ, Peng C, Son JH. 2003. Oxidative stress regulated genes in nigral dopaminergic neuronal cells: correlation with the known pathology in Parkinson's disease. Brain Res Mol Brain Res   110(1): 76-84.

You S-A, Archacki SR. Angheloiu G, Moravee CS,Rao S, Kinter M, Topol, EJ, Wang Q. 2003. Proteomic approach to coronary atherosclerosis shows ferritin light chain as a significant marker: evidence consistent with the iron hypothesis in atherosclerosis. Physiol Genomics. 13:25-30.

Youdim MB, Ben-Shachar D, Riederer P. 1989. Is Parkinson's disease a progressive siderosis of substantia nigra resulting in iron and melanin induced neurodegeneration? Acta Neurol Scand Suppl. 126:47-54.

———— 1990. The role of monoamine oxidase, iron-melanin interaction, and intracellular calcium in Parkinson's disease. J Neural Transm Suppl. 32:239-48.

———— 1991. Iron in brain function and dysfunction with emphasis on Parkinson's disease. Eur Neurol. 31 Suppl 1:34-40.

Youdim MB, Riederer P. 1993. The role of iron in senescence of dopamiergic neurons in Parkinson's disease. J Neural Transm Suppl. 40:57-67.

Youdim MB, Ben-Schachar D, Riederer P. 1993. The possible role of iron in the etiopathology of Parkinson's disease. Mov Disord. 8(1):1-12.

Youdim MB, Ben-Shachar D, Eshel G, Finberg JP, Riederer P. 1993. The neurotoxicity of iron and nitric oxide. Relevance to the etiology of Parkinson's disease. Adv Neurol. 60:259-66.

Youdim MB. 2003. What we have learnt from CDNA microarray gene expression studies about the role of iron in MPTP induced neurodegeneration and Parkinson's disease? J Neural Transm Suppl. (65):73-88.

Youdim MB, Stephenson G, Ben-Shachar D. 2004. Ironing iron out in Parkinson's disease and other neurodegenerative diseases with iron chelators: a lesson from 6-hydroxydopamine and iron chelators, desferal and VK-28. Ann N Y Acad Sci. 1012:306-25.

Youdim MB, Fridkin M, Zheng H. 2004. Novel bifunctional drugs targeting monoamine oxidase inhibition and iron chelation as an approach to neuroprotection in Parkinson's disease and other neurodegenerative diseases. J Neural Transm. 111:1455-71.

Youdim MB, Fridkin M, Zheng H. 2005. Bifunctional drug derivatives of MAO-B inhibitor rasagiline and iron chelator VK-28 as a more effective approach to treatment of brain ageing in ageing neurodegenerative diseases. Mech Ageing Dev. 126:317-26.

Yu Z, Eaton JW, Persson HL. 2003. The radioprotective agent, amifostine, suppresses the reactivity of intralysosomal iron. 8(6):347-55.

Zacharski LR, Ornstein DL, Woloshin S, Schwartz LM. 2000. Association of age, sex, and race with body iron stores in adults: analysis of NHANES III data. Am Heart J. 140(1):98-104.

Zafar AM, Zuberi L, Khan AH, Ahsan H. 2007. Utility of MRI in assessment of pituitary iron overload. Pak Med Assoc. 57(9):475-7.

Zecca L, Youdim MBH, Riederer P, Conner JR, Crichton, RR. 2004. Iron, brain ageing and neurodegenerative disorders. Nature Reviews Neuroscience. 5:863-73.

Zhong JL, Yiakouvaki A, Patricia H, Tyrrell RM, Pourzand. 2004. Susceptibility of skin cells to UVA-induced necrotic cell death reflects the intracellular level of labile iron. J Invest Dermatol. 123:771-80.

Zhou JR, Erdman JW Jr. 1995. Phytic acid in health and disease. Crit Rev Food Sci Nutr. 35(6):495-508.

Zucca FA, Bellei C, Gianelli S, Terreni MR, Gallorini M, Rizzio G, Albertini A, Zecca L. 2006. Neuromelanin and iron in human locus coeruleus and substantia nigra during aging: consequences for neuronal vulnerability. J Neural Transm. 113(6):757-67.

Index

Made in the USA
Columbia, SC
20 May 2024

35983149R00140